Pharmacology

Pharmacology

Josephine Randall

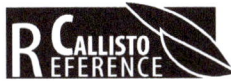

R CALLISTO REFERENCE

www.callistoreference.com

Callisto Reference,
118-35 Queens Blvd., Suite 400,
Forest Hills, NY 11375, USA

Visit us on the World Wide Web at:
www.callistoreference.com

ISBN: 978-1-64116-542-6 (Hardback)

Cataloging-in-Publication Data

Pharmacology / Josephine Randall.
    p. cm.
Includes bibliographical references and index.
ISBN 978-1-64116-542-6
1. Pharmacology. 2. Drugs. 3. Pharmacy. 4. Developmental pharmacology.
5. Pharmacology, Experimental. I. Randall, Josephine.
RM301 .P43 2022
615.1--dc23

Table of Contents

Preface

It is with great pleasure that I present this book. It has been carefully written after numerous discussions with my peers and other practitioners of the field. I would like to take this opportunity to thank my family and friends who have been extremely supporting at every step in my life.

Pharmacology is a branch of pharmaceutical sciences that focuses on the study of drug action and medication action. It studies the interactions between a living organism and chemicals that affect the biochemical function. Pharmacology includes drug design and synthesis, drug composition and properties, molecular and cellular mechanisms, molecular diagnostics, chemical biology, organ mechanisms, therapy, medical applications and antipathogenic capabilities. Pharmacodynamics and pharmacokinetics are two main branches of pharmacology. Pharmacodynamics studies how a drug influences the biological systems. Pharmacokinetics studies the effects of biological systems on a drug. The absorption, metabolism, distribution and excretion of chemicals from the biological systems are also studied under this field. This book unfolds the innovative aspects of pharmacology which will be crucial for the progress of this field in the future. Some of the diverse topics covered herein address the varied branches that fall under this category. Through this book, we attempt to further enlighten the readers about the new concepts in this field.

The chapters below are organized to facilitate a comprehensive understanding of the subject:

Chapter – Introduction

The biological branch which is concerned with the study of drug or medication action is referred to as pharmacology. It focuses on the interactions between living organisms and the chemicals which affect normal or abnormal biochemical function. The topics elaborated in this chapter will help in gaining a better perspective about pharmacology as well as its importance in the field of dentistry.

Chapter – Drugs in Pharmacology

Any substance that causes a change in the physiology or psychology of an organism when consumed is known as a drug. Various areas of study related to drugs are drug class, drug discovery, drug development, drug delivery, drug detoxification, drug interaction, etc. This chapter discusses in detail these processes and concepts related to drugs.

Chapter – Pharmacokinetics

Pharmacokinetics is the branch of pharmacology which is concerned with determining the fate of the substances administered to a living organism. This chapter discusses in detail various aspects of pharmacokinetics including the absorption, distribution, metabolism and elimination of pharmaceutical drugs.

Chapter – Pharmacodynamics

Pharmacodynamics refers to the study of the physiologic and biochemical effects of drugs. This chapter has been carefully written to provide an easy understanding of the varied facets of pharmacodynamics such as dose-response relationship, Schild regression and pharmacodynamics modeling.

Chapter – Psychopharmacology

The scientific study of the effects of drugs on sensation, mood, thinking and behavior is known as psychopharmacology. Some of the psychoactive drugs which are studied within this field are psychiatric medication, benzodiazepine and hallucinogens. All these diverse drugs as well as the role of psychopharmacology in mental health have been carefully analyzed in this chapter.

Chapter – Diverse Fields in Pharmacology

There are various related fields of pharmacology. A few of them are pharmacoepidemiology, pharmacotoxicology, medicinal chemistry, pharmacogenomics and pharmacoinformatics. These diverse related fields of pharmacology have been thoroughly discussed in this chapter.

Josephine Randall

1

Introduction

The biological branch which is concerned with the study of drug or medication action is referred to as pharmacology. It focuses on the interactions between living organisms and the chemicals which affect normal or abnormal biochemical function. The topics elaborated in this chapter will help in gaining a better perspective about pharmacology as well as its importance in the field of dentistry.

PHARMACOLOGY

Pharmacology is the branch of medicine concerned with the uses, effects and modes of action of drugs. Drugs are defined as chemical substances that have an effect on living organisms; medicines are drugs used to prevent or treat disease. The administration route, health and age of the patient, and the chemical structure of the drug all play a role in how fast it will act. A drug is considered effective if it elicits the desired therapeutic response with minimal side effects.

All drugs elicit more than one response and the use of multiple drugs at the same time may lead to desirable or dangerous drug interactions. Fortunately, due to effective drug control laws, the desired therapeutic response usually occurs and the side effects of most official drugs are predictable, minimal and can be reduced by adjusting the dose of the drug. That being said, a few patients experience side effects strong enough to warrant discontinuing the drug treatment regime. Unlike most side effects, systemic allergic reactions are unpredictable and while most result in hives some cause respiratory distress, vascular collapse, and death. Interactions between multiple drugs taken concurrently may result in either an increase or decrease of one or both drugs due to changes in each drug's absorption, distribution, metabolism, or excretion (ADME) characteristics. The majority of drug interactions are known and can be prevented by checking the appropriate data base. Patients taking any form of drug should be monitored for side effects, systemic allergic reactions, and drug interactions (if taking more than one drug).

Drug Classifications

Drugs fall into two distinct categories: Those that require a physician's prescription to obtain (Rx) and those that can be purchased over the counter (OTC); both are regulated by the United States Food and Drug Administration (FDA).

Within these categories they are further classified by the body system they effect, how they are used, or how they elicit their response. Drugs may be referred to by their chemical names, official names, brand names, or by their generic names. Because it describes the drug's exact molecular structure the chemical name is complex and really only useful to chemists. Upon approval the FDA gives each drug an official name. Trademark or brand names are proprietary and assigned and registered by the drug's manufacturer. In order to distinguish them from generic names, official drug names and brand names are capitalized when in print. The generic name is non-proprietary, simpler, and not capitalized when in print.

How Drugs Work

Most drugs act by forming chemical bonds with specific receptor sites within the body to stimulate or inhibit a response. While drugs alter the body's physiologic activity along existing chemical pathways, they do not create new pathways or responses. The success of a drug's response depends on two factors: its molecular fit and the number of receptor sites it bonds to. The better the fit and the greater number of receptor sites occupied, the stronger the response. Chemical agonists fit and bond well into receptor sites and therefore elicit a strong response. Partial chemical agonists bond but only fit well enough to elicit a partial response. Chemical antagonists also bond to receptor sites but do not fit well enough to elicit a response; their main role is to occupy the site and prevent agonists from bonding. If a receptor site is occupied other drugs cannot bond to it.

In order for drugs elicit a response they must first be dissolved in the patient's blood or plasma and then transported to their respective receptor sites. Once dissolved, they go thorough four distinct stages: absorption, distribution, metabolism, and excretion (ADME).

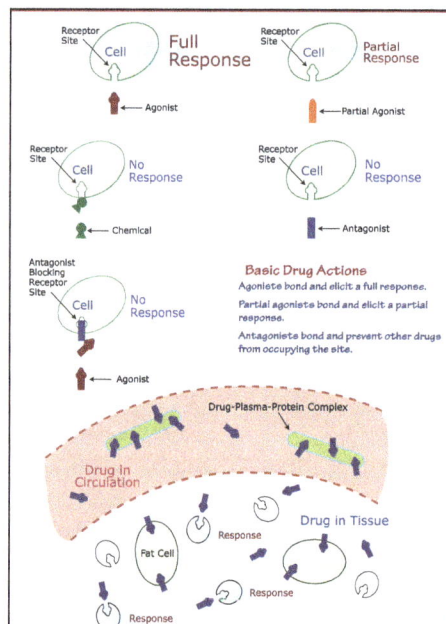

Enzymes produced by the liver are the body's primary way of breaking down drugs and preparing them for removal (metabolism). Once inactivated, drug metabolites—and in some cases the active drug—are excreted from the body primarily through the urinary system and kidneys. Other less utilized removal methods are via the GI tract (bile), lungs (exhalation), and skin. Age, disease, smoking, and dehydration may decrease liver and renal function slowing both drug metabolism and excretion.

Absorption is the process by which a drug is transported from its administration site into general circulation. The rate of absorption depends on the patient's hydration status, the administration route, the blood flow through the tissue at the administration site, and the solubility of the drug. Once absorbed most drugs bind to—and are carried by—plasma proteins in the blood and lymph for distribution. When bound, the large size of the resulting drug/protein complex prevent the drug from crossing the vascular membranes into the tissue; and a drug must cross into tissue to bathe receptor sites, become metabolized by the liver, or be excreted by the kidneys. Furthermore, once in the extra cellular space, fat soluble drugs are likely to bind to fat cells rendering them temporarily inactive. As serum drug levels change due to a drug response, metabolism, or excretion, molecules of the bound drug are released from the drug/protein complex and/or fat cells to maintain the equilibrium between the free and bound drug. It is only the unbound drug in solution that is pharmacologically active. The amount of the drug that reaches the receptor sites determines the strength of its response. Serum levels of the drug must remain within a specific range in order to render the desired therapeutic effect.

Drug Administration in a Wilderness Environment

Drugs are administered by one of three routes: through the digestive system via ingestion, directly into the body's fluid reservoir via injection, and through body membranes via the lungs, mucous membranes, or skin. Choosing and administering a drug in a wilderness context by non-physicians should be done only in specific circumstances and according to protocols established by the expedition's—or organization's—physician advisor. Hydration, even in healthy people, is always a concern in a wilderness environment and becomes even more so when administering drugs. Because dehydration equals poor absorption, distribution, metabolism, and excretion (ADME) and inhibits the desired therapeutic response, make sure that your patient is well-hydrated before administrating any drugs. Because oral drugs are effective, easy to carry, and simple to administer, they tend to make up the majority of the drugs carried in an expedition first aid kit. Before an oral medication can reach general circulation it must survive the acids and enzymes of the digestive system, be successfully transported across the stomach or intestinal lining, and survive the initial pass through the liver. Throughout the process hydration is extremely important; even in a well-hydrated patient oral medications should be given with water (8 ounce minimum).

The skin and mucous membranes are another common drug administration route used in a wilderness setting because, like oral drugs, they are effective, easy to carry, and simple to administer. Ear and eye drops are used to treat local infections. Rectal suppositories are used to treat constipation and nausea. Vaginal suppositories or creams are used to treat vaginitis. Topical skin ointments are used to treat local allergic reactions, promote healing in partial thickness wounds, and treat a variety of cutaneous fungal infections. Sub-lingual or buccal glucose tablets are used to treat hypoglycemia in the insulin dependant diabetic and sub-lingual tablets are used to treat angina.

Absorption via inhalation is influenced by the depth of the patient's respirations. Absorption in the lungs is more effective when a spacer is used to disperse the medication prior to inhalation and the patient can take a deep breath and hold the drug in their lungs for a few seconds before exhaling. In a wilderness setting the inhalation route tends to be reserved for participants suffering from asthma.

While all types of injections bypass the digestive system and frequently offer the fastest absorption and distribution route, they should not be the first choice for a expedition first aid kit because they are expensive, difficult to carry, and require advanced training to use. Subcutaneous (SC) and intramuscular (IM) injections of epinephrine are commonly given—primarily by auto-injectors—to treat systemic allergic reactions. Because there are more blood vessels in muscles than in subcutaneous tissue, absorption is faster via IM injection. Give IM injections in the belly of the muscle where blood flow is the greatest and there are no large arteries or veins; the most common site used in the field is the anterior thigh.

Infusions are similar to injections in that they are an invasive procedure requiring a needle; however, during infusions the needle—or a catheter— remains in place for hours and occasionally days.

Intravenous (IV) infusions provide the most direct route to the blood and are commonly used in the acute pre-hospital setting where large amounts of fluid are required. Subcutaneous (SC) infusions are easier to start, maintain, have significantly less problems and potential problems than other infusion methods, and may be of value in the marine environment when used to treat dehydration secondary to sea sickness (hypodermoclysis). Intraosseous (IO) or bone infusions are similar to IVs in that they require specialized equipment and training but are easier to use in hazardous environments. Infusion solutions and kits are rarely carried in the backcountry due their relatively high weight, low need, storage problems, difficulty of administration in challenging environments, and the high level of training needed to administer them correctly even under the best of circumstances. As a result, infusions tend to be reserved for inbound rescue teams, remote field clinics who are staffed with field paramedics, nurses, or physicians, and have the capacity to carry or store the necessary equipment.

When choosing a drug, make sure that you:

- Have authorization,
- Adhere to your protocols,

- Review the patient's history for prior systemic allergic reactions to the drug,

- Make sure there is no possibility of dangerous drug interactions if multiple drugs are to be given,

- Review and advise the patient of the possible side effects.

Prior to administration, assess and document the patient's response to any prior medications and make sure they are hydrated. Make sure you have the:

- Right patient,

- Right drug,

- Right administration route,

- Right dose,

- Right time.

After administering the drug, document all of the above in the patient's soap note and/or a separate drug log.

Herbs

Medicinal herbs have been successfully used to treat ailments for thousands of years. Their gathering, preparation, and use have been documented in the writings and folklore of numerous cultures worldwide. Their use has been refined by generations and provides a built-in safety factor unavailable in modern drugs. Although herbs may be evaluated according to their pharmacological actions and chemical compounds, the constituents of the entire plant are greater than the sum of its parts. Some plant components are synergistic and enhance the herb's action far beyond the synthesized "active" compound, while other constituents buffer chemicals that would, without their presence, cause harmful side-effects. In addition to their direct therapeutic affect many medicinal herbs provide necessary trace elements and vitamins required for effective healing. Pharmaceutically both herbs and drugs are chemicals and work within the body in a similar manner; although, the line between therapeutic and toxic doses tends to be much broader with herbs thus increasing their safety factor when used by lay people. Herbs may be gathered and stored for use as the dried herb, dried powders, essential oils, tinctures, ointments, liniments, capsules, lozenges, and syrups. Teas may be made from fresh or dried herbs, tinctures, and tonics.

- Essential oils extracted from the plant are used as inhalants and when diluted, for massage; they should not be taken internally.

- Fresh herbs steeped in alcohol or cider vinegar produce concentrated tinctures. Tinctures are taken internally or used to make teas, compresses, or ointments. Be aware, some herbs, like comfrey, should not be taken internally. A single tincture made from multiple herbs is referred to as a tonic. Unless you are a trained herbalist or have done your research, take care in mixing herbs. Different herbs taken together—like different drugs—can be either synergistic and amplify their effects, nullify one another, or produce an unexpected and potentially dangerous side effect.

- Infusions are teas made from the flowers and leaves of fresh or dried herbs. To make an infusion pour boiling water over the herb, cover, and allow it to steep for 10-15 minutes before straining. Infusions reserve the volatile oils present in the herb.

- Decoctions are teas made by boiling the hard, woody parts of an herb. The roots, woody stems, bark, or nuts are first chopped (or ground) and then boiled for 10-15 minutes before straining.

- Compresses are made by soaking a clean cloth in an infusion or decoction. Poultices are similar to compresses but are made by wrapping the herb in gauze before applying to the skin. Both compresses and poultices are applied hot to the injured area and changed when they become cool. The active components are absorbed through the skin.

- Ointments are made by combining the fresh herb or tincture with a base of wax, fat, or oil that is then applied to the skin.

- Liniments are an oil based herbal extract and used externally.

- Capsules are gelatin containers filled with powdered herbs or oils.

- Lozenges are powdered herbs or oil combined with gum or dried sugar.

- Syrups are tinctures added to sugar.

Herbs may be carried and stored in chopped or powdered form for later use in infusions, decoctions, compresses, or poultices. Since they do not keep well, water-based infusions and decoctions should be used immediately. Essential oils, ointments, liniments, and tinctures are prepared prior to use and for specific purposes; they are easily carried and last for years.

MECHANISM OF ACTION

The term mechanism of action is a pharmacological term that you commonly hear associated with medications or drugs. Let's gain an understanding of what mechanism of action means, and provide examples within the context of health conditions.

Mechanism of action refers to the biochemical process through which a drug produces its effect. Drugs bind to receptors, which are located on the surface of cells or within a cell's cytoplasm — a jelly-like substance within a cell.

When bound, the drug can act as either an agonist or an antagonist. Agonist drugs activate the receptors they bind to, which either increases or decreases activity within the cell. Antagonist drugs, on the other hand, block the receptors so that natural agonists within the body cannot bind.

Most drugs bind to a specific type of receptor, and this term is called receptor selectivity. The ability of a drug to bind to a certain receptor is based on its unique chemical structure.

The mechanism of action of a medication is the specific biological process through which the medication causes the reduction in symptoms. For example, the mechanism of action of selective serotonin reuptake inhibitors, or SSRIs, is well known. SSRIs inhibit the reuptake of serotonin. This increases the level of serotonin in the brain, which improves a person's mood.

For some drugs, the mechanism of action is unknown — so the drug works, but scientists are not sure exactly how it creates its therapeutic effect. An example of a medication with an unknown mechanism of action is lithium, a mood stabilizer used in the treatment of bipolar disorder. Other drugs have multiple known mechanisms of action, like caffeine.

Sometimes the term mechanism of action is used to describe a non-drug treatment. For example, the mechanism of action of a psychosocial intervention — like psychotherapy — is the specific intervention that produces a change in a patient's symptoms. Experts propose that the mechanism of action of psychotherapy is based on the patient-therapist interaction, and how actively they participate in sessions.

IMPORTANCE OF PHARMACOLOGY IN DENTISTRY

Pharmacology plays an important role in dentistry. The aim of dental pharmacology is to understand the scientific aspects of how drugs used in dentistry act within various body systems.

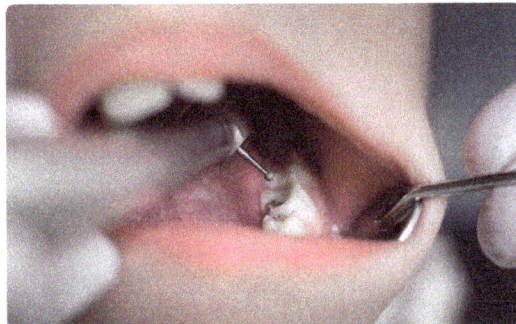

Pharmacology encompasses two aspects of drug metabolism – pharmacokinetics and pharmacodynamics. While pharmacokinetics deals with drug absorption, distribution, metabolism, and excretion, pharmacodynamics deals with drug efficacy, safety, receptor occupancy (potency), and drug interactions. Knowledge of all these aspects with respect to a given drug is necessary in order to successfully treat a dental condition using the drug.

Pharmacokinetics

Following the oral or topical administration of a drug, its absorption requires that it be lipid soluble, as it can then diffuse through the epithelium and reach the capillaries.

Drug molecules travel in the bloodstream either in the free or unbound state, or bound to plasma proteins. Only the unbound drug is free and is distributed to the tissues. Further, the parent drug may be converted to a number of metabolites.

Either the parent drugs or their metabolites may be active/inactive and toxic/non-toxic. After metabolism, the course of elimination of the drug also varies depending on the route of administration and the physicochemical properties of the drug.

Pharmacodynamics

Drug action depends on the state of the receptors (active or inactive). Drugs interact with receptors in a variety of ways. Antagonists bind to receptors and do not activate either receptor state. Agonists bind as well as activate the receptors. Inverse agonists selectively stimulate the inactive receptor state by initiating the cellular response opposite to that generated by a natural agonist.

The efficacy and potency of drugs used in dentistry is determined by how well the drug binds with the receptors and triggers the desired response. The potency of these drugs is determined as the amount of drug required to produce a chosen intensity of effect. The drug doses are calculated for a given formulation (spray, gargle, rinse, tablet, ointment, or patch etc.) on the basis of all these factors. Additionally, it is equally important to understand the toxic effects associated with dental medicines, and any interactions with other drugs.

Medications used in Dentistry

Several classes of drugs are utilized in dentistry depending on the requirement.

For instance, local anesthetics, general anesthetics, or nitrous oxide are administered to reduce the perception of pain associated with several dental conditions and procedures, and accompanying anxiety. Anesthetic medications bind to the sodium channels, blocking the conduction of nerve stimuli, and hence they are useful during procedures such as tooth extraction.

Local anesthetic ointments are also prescribed for application before meals, in order to numb the area of pain, so that the patient can eat peacefully. The onset and duration of action of these medications depend upon factors such as proximity to target site, concentration (dose), pH of the tissue, lipid/aqueous solubility, protein binding, and tissue redistribution of the drug. Their side effects may range from mild confusion and talkativeness to tonic-clonic seizures and severe depression. Nerve injury is also one of the serious but less common adverse effects of dental anesthetics.

Anti-inflammatory and analgesic medications including corticosteroids are also used to relieve the pain. These are the most common categories of drugs used in dentistry, and are available in different dosage forms. Analgesics such as non-steroidal anti-inflammatory drugs (NSAIDs) attach themselves to cyclooxygenase (COX) receptors – COX1 or COX2, and inhibit these enzymes. They possess antipyretic and anti-inflammatory activities in addition to analgesic activities. COX2 inhibitors are particularly beneficial as they produce fewer or no gastrointestinal adverse effects compared with COX1 inhibitors. Other side effects of NSAIDs include renotoxicity, dyspepsia, and anaphylactic reactions. Opioids are another category of drugs used in dentistry as analgesics and sedatives. They directly affect the central nervous system. Addiction and withdrawal symptoms are potential problems associated with the long-term usage of opioids.

Another important category is antibiotics and antiseptics which are employed to treat the ailments such as plaque and gingivitis, and anti-fungal medicines which are used to treat oral thrush. These medicines target the gums and the dental roots, and are available as oral pills, mouth rinses and gargles. They are also utilized to treat breath odor. Bacteriostatic as well as bactericidal antibiotics include penicillins, cephalosporins, tetracyclines, aminoglycosides etc. classes of drugs. The choice of antibiotics is driven by several factors including type of infection, age of the patient, compliance, medical history, concomitant medications, and bacterial resistance.

Also, fluoride containing products are used to prevent tooth decay on a non-prescription basis in areas without fluoridation of water.

IMPACT OF PHARMACOLOGY ON A SOCIETY

Pharmacology is one of the focal points of modern science and research activities. It seems that in the modern, high developed world all drugs and medicine are already invented and produced, but the up-to date realities and scientific achievements cause improvements of existing medicaments and creation of new efficient pharmaceutical substances. At the same time more and more often the humanity faces the mutated strains of different viruses, various serious epidermis and fatal diseases.

Thus, there are a lot of thought questions and urgent problems that should be considered and solved by the best scientists in the field of pharmacology. Biomedical scientists make their efforts to examine body functioning and drug influence on a human to reduce side effects that can be caused by taking medicine and improve obtained results in disease treatment. Interdisciplinary links and advanced technologies give a helping hand in gaining the best and the most efficient outcome.

2

Drugs in Pharmacology

Any substance that causes a change in the physiology or psychology of an organism when consumed is known as a drug. Various areas of study related to drugs are drug class, drug discovery, drug development, drug delivery, drug detoxification, drug interaction, etc. This chapter discusses in detail these processes and concepts related to drugs.

A drug is a substance used to prevent or cure a disease or ailment or to alleviate its symptoms. In the U.S. some drugs are available over-the-counter while others can be purchased only with a doctor's prescription. Drugs can be taken orally, via a skin patch, by injection, or via an inhaler, to name the most common methods.

The pharmaceutical industry, which is concerned with the development and marketing of drugs, is a key component of the health sector, which is the most profitable industry in the U.S. economy at an estimated $24.4 billion in revenues in 2018.

Development of new and improved drugs, or pharmaceuticals, is a complex and costly business in the U.S. Some of the biggest American corporations, such as Johnson & Johnson, Pfizer, Merck, and Eli Lilly, are in in the business of researching, testing, manufacturing and marketing new drugs.

In addition, biotechnology has evolved in recent years as a major new branch of the drug business. Biotechnology companies concentrate on research and development of new cures based on genetic manipulation. The big players in the field include Amgen, Gilead Sciences, and Celgene Corp.

In the United States, prescription drugs must be approved by the Food and Drug Administration (FDA). The agency's Center for Drug Evaluation and Research (CDER) acts as a consumer watchdog.

How Drugs get to Market

On average, it takes about 10 years and costs about $2.6 billion for a new drug to make it from its initial discovery to a doctor's office, according to an industry group. The process has five main phases:

- Development and discovery
- Preclinical research

- Clinical research

- FDA review

- Post-market safety monitoring

In the development and discovery phase, researchers explore new possibilities. They may investigate unexpected effects of existing drugs, test new molecular compounds, or create new technologies that allow drugs to work differently in the body.

In the preclinical research phase, when a potential new drug is identified, researchers determine the correct dosages and methods of administration, side effects, interactions with other drugs, and effectiveness. They also study the drug's absorption, metabolization, and excretion characteristics.

In the clinical research phase, the company first tests the substance in the lab, or "in vitro," and sometimes on animals, or "in vivo." Depending on the outcome, the drug may then be tested on human subjects in clinical trials to determine whether it is safe and effective. A drug that passes that hurdle is submitted to the CDER for review. The agency employs pharmacologists, chemists, statisticians, physicians, and other scientists who conduct an independent and unbiased review of the drug and the documentation submitted with it. That process typically takes six to 10 months to complete. The drug company will be allowed to sell the drug if the CDER determines that the drug's benefits outweigh its risks. It is then responsible for monitoring reports on the drug's effectiveness and unanticipated side effects.

Name Brand vs. Generic Drugs

Drugs sold in the U.S. may be name-brand or generic. A name-brand drug can be patented for 20 years after its discovery or invention. Once the patent expires, other manufacturers can produce and market generic equivalents of that drug.

Generic equivalents are increasingly prescribed as they become available in the U.S. because of their relatively low cost. Generics are required to have the same medicinal ingredients, and therefore the same therapeutic effects, to receive FDA approval for sale as substitutes.

MEDICATION

A medication is a substance that is taken into or placed on the body that does one of the following things:

- Most medications are used to cure a disease or condition. For example, antibiotics are given to cure an infection.

- Medications are also given to treat a medical condition. For example, anti-depressants are given to treat depression.

- Medications are also given to relieve symptoms of an illness. For example, pain relievers are given to reduce pain.

- Vaccinations are given to prevent diseases. For example, the Flu Vaccine helps to prevent the person from complications of having the flu.

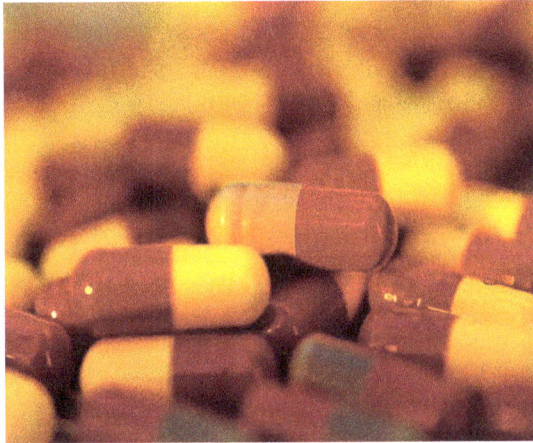

How do Medications Work?

Medications get into the body in a number of different ways. The way the medication enters the body is called the "route".

The most common "route" for medications is orally (by mouth) in the form of pills, capsules or liquids.

However, if the person is unable to take medications in this way, or if the medication is not available in oral form, medications can enter the body by other routes.

Here are some of the different routes:

- Oral medications are taken by mouth, in pill, capsule or liquid form, they are swallowed and pass into the digestive system. The medications are then broken down in either the stomach or the intestines and are absorbed in the same way as food. They then pass through the liver before entering the bloodstream. Once a medication enters the bloodstream, it circulates to the site where its action is needed.

- Nasal (into the nose), buccal (placed in the cheek) and sublingual (placed under the tongue) medications are absorbed through the thin mucous membrane that lines the inside of the nose and mouth and enters the bloodstream in this way.

- Eye drops and ear drops are applied directly and are typically used to treat specific problems or symptoms within the eye or the ear. However, some eye drops, such as those used to treat glaucoma, can be absorbed into the bloodstream.

- Transdermal (through the skin) medications are applied to the skin either by patch or in creams or lotions and pass through the skin into the blood vessels.

- Topical medications can be applied directly to the skin and tend to have a very localized effect. They do not usually enter the bloodstream in significant amounts.

- Subcutaneous medications are injected into the fatty tissue just below the skin and travel from the fatty tissue into the bloodstream.

- Enteral medications, those given through a G tube or a J tube go directly into the stomach or intestine and pass into the digestive system and then through the liver and into the bloodstream. Some medications that are given by mouth cannot be given via G tube or J tube. Always routinely check with the pharmacist about this.

- Rectal and vaginal medications, such as suppositories, enemas and creams are inserted into the rectum or the vagina and absorbed by the blood vessels in the rectal or vaginal wall.

- Inhaled medications have a direct effect on the lungs.

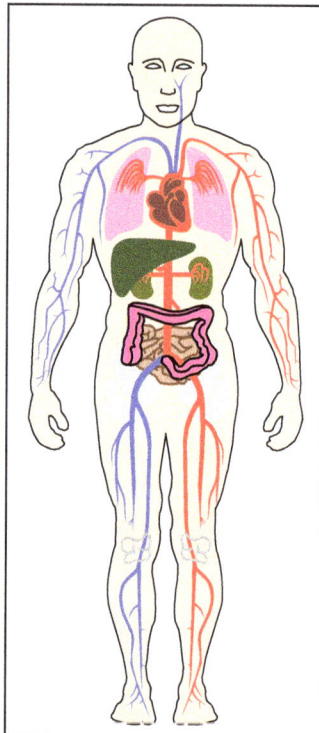

Medication Effects

Local Effect: Some medications, such as eye drops or topical skin creams or ointments, are applied directly to the area that needs treatment.

These applications tend to have a very localized effect and do not usually enter the bloodstream in significant quantities.

For example: Antibiotic ointment is applied to a scrape on the skin. The ointment stays on the surface of the skin, where the medication effect is needed.

Systemic Effect: Some medications, such as pills or liquids given orally, rectal suppositories, Transdermal patches and subcutaneous injections end up in the bloodstream and act on a specific organ or system within the body.

These medications are said to have a systemic effect. For example, anti-depressant medications taken orally are circulated through the bloodstream and work by increasing the amount of certain chemicals in the brain.

DRUG CLASS

A drug class is a term used to describe medications that are grouped together because of their similarity. There are four dominant methods of classifying these groups:

- By their therapeutic use, meaning the types of condition they are used to treat.

- By their mechanism of action, meaning the specific biochemical reaction that occurs when you take a drug.

- By their mode of action, meaning the specific way in which the body responds to a drug.

- By their chemical structure.

Based on these diverse classification methods, some drugs may be grouped together under one system but not another. In other cases, a drug may have multiple uses or actions (such as the drug finasteride, which is used to treat an enlarged prostate and regrow hair) and may be included in multiple drug classes within a single classification system.

This doesn't even take into account the drugs that are used off-label for reasons other than what they were approved. A prime example is a levothyroxine which is approved to treat hypothyroidism (low thyroid function) but is often used off-label to treat depression.

As newer and more advanced drugs are being introduced into the market each year— including next-generation targeted therapies, gene therapies, and personalized medicines—the classification of drugs will likely become even more diverse and distinct, reflecting our ever-expanding knowledge about human biochemistry as a whole.

Purpose of Drug Classification

The aim of drug classification is to ensure that you use a drug safely to achieve the utmost benefit. Ultimately, every time you take a drug, your body chemistry is altered. While this effect is meant to be therapeutic, it can also cause side effects that may be harmful. Moreover, if you take multiple drugs, your body chemistry may be changed in such a way that a drug is far less effective or the side effects are far more severe.

By noting the classification of a drug, you and your doctor can have a better understanding of what to expect when you take it, what the risks are, and which drugs you can switch to if needed. This designation also helps identify drug-drug interactions and the potential for drug resistance and ensures the appropriate staging of treatment.

Drug-Drug Interactions

The effectiveness of a drug can often be reduced if the action of one drug diminishes the action of another. Since drugs are commonly classified by their mode and mechanism of action, any interaction affecting one drug will usually affect drugs of the same class, either by interfering with their absorption or the way in which the body metabolizes the drug.

For example, antacids invariably work by blocking stomach acid but, by doing so, deplete the stomach of the acids needed to break down and absorb a class of HIV drug known as protease inhibitors. If the medications are taken together, the HIV drug will be less able to control the viral infection.

Similarly, many classes of drug are cleared from the body by a liver enzyme called CYP3A4. If you take two drugs that are each metabolized by the enzyme, the drugs may not be cleared as effectively and begin to build up, leading to toxicity. By classifying a drug by its CYP3A4 action, doctors are better able to avoid this interaction.

The same applies to drugs like methotrexate and Advil (ibuprofen) that are metabolized by the kidneys. Their concurrent use may not only lead to toxicity but kidney failure. Other classes of the drug need to be used with caution when combined with those that affect the same organ system.

For example, non-steroidal anti-inflammatory drugs (NSAIDs) like Motrin or aspirin are often avoided when taking anticoagulants (blood thinners) like warfarin, as the former can increase the risk of bleeding while the latter inhibits the clotting of blood. It is for this same reason that two NSAIDs are not combined. In some cases, doubling the class of drug only serves to double the risk or severity of the side effects.

Drug Resistance

Medications used to treat chronic infections do so in a specific way. If used incorrectly or for a long period of time, a drug may lose its potency as the infection becomes resistant to its effects. If this occurs, other drugs of the same class may also fail or not work as well.

Antibiotics (of which there are seven major classes) and HIV drugs (of which there are six classes) are two such examples. Depending on the class, some may have a greater potential for resistance than others. To better overcome resistance, multiple classes are commonly prescribed to achieve optimal control of the bacterial or viral infection.

Treatment Staging

Drugs are often staged so that you are first exposed to over-the-counter drugs with the fewest side effects and then moved to prescription options that have more serious side effects. The drugs are often staged by the class under a prescribed guideline, with preferred classes used for first-line therapies and alternate classes used for subsequent therapies.

For example, when treating severe pain, doctors will generally use over-the-counter NSAIDs first and prescription NSAIDs second before moving onto highly addictive, Schedule II opioid drugs like Oxycontin (oxycodone) and Vicodin (hydrocodone).

Drug staging is also vital to treating chronic diseases like diabetes, hypertension, chronic obstructive pulmonary disease (COPD), and autoimmune disorders like rheumatoid arthritis. In cases like these, the class of drug typically directs the appropriate staging of treatment.

ATC Classification System

In the end, there are numerous ways to classify a drug and thousands of different drug classes and subclasses. To bring order to chaos, in 1976 the World Health Organization (WHO) created a multi-dimensional system called the Anatomical Therapeutic Chemical (ATC) Classification System, which categorizes a drug based on five levels:

- Level One: Describes the organ system the drug treats.

- Level Two: Describes the drug's therapeutic effect.

- Level Three: Describes the mechanism/mode of action.

- Level Four: Describes the general chemical properties of the drug.

- Level Five: Describes the chemical components that make up the drug (essentially the chemical name of the drug, such as finasteride or ibuprofen).

For each level, either a letter or numbers are assigned. While not useful for the consumer, the ATC system is able to classify the active ingredient of a drug under a strict hierarchy so that it is appropriately used and not mistaken for another drug.

DRUG DISCOVERY

In the fields of medicine, biotechnology and pharmacology, drug discovery is the process by which new candidate medications are discovered.

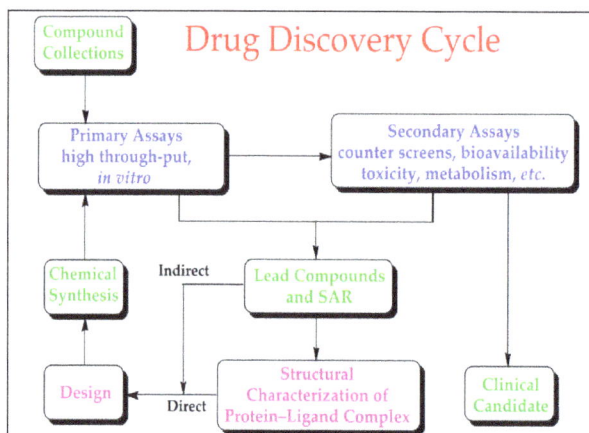

Historically, drugs were discovered by identifying the active ingredient from traditional remedies or by serendipitous discovery, as with penicillin. More recently, chemical libraries of synthetic small molecules, natural products or extracts were screened in intact cells or whole organisms to identify substances that had a desirable therapeutic effect in a process known as classical pharmacology. After sequencing of the human genome allowed rapid cloning and synthesis of large quantities of purified proteins, it has become common practice to use high throughput screening of large compounds libraries against isolated biological targets which are hypothesized to be disease-modifying in a process known as reverse pharmacology. Hits from these screens are then tested in cells and then in animals for efficacy.

Modern drug discovery involves the identification of screening hits, medicinal chemistry and optimization of those hits to increase the affinity, selectivity (to reduce the potential of side effects), efficacy/potency, metabolic stability (to increase the half-life), and oral bioavailability. Once a compound that fulfills all of these requirements has been identified, the process of drug development can continue, and, if successful, clinical trials. One or more of these steps may, but not necessarily, involve computer-aided drug design.

Modern drug discovery is thus usually a capital-intensive process that involves large investments by pharmaceutical industry corporations as well as national governments (who provide grants and loan guarantees). Despite advances in technology and understanding of biological systems, drug discovery is still a lengthy, "expensive, difficult, and inefficient process" with low rate of new therapeutic discovery. In 2010, the research and development cost of each new molecular entity was about US$1.8 billion. Currently, basic discovery research is funded primarily by governments and by philanthropic organizations, while late-stage development is funded primarily by pharmaceutical companies or venture capitalists. To be allowed to come to market, drugs must undergo several phases of clinical trials, and most drugs fail. Small companies have a critical role, often then selling the rights to larger companies that have the resources to run the clinical trials.

Discovering drugs that may be a commercial success, or a public health success, involves a complex interaction between investors, industry, academia, patent laws, regulatory exclusivity, marketing and the need to balance secrecy with communication. Meanwhile, for disorders whose rarity means that no large commercial success or public health effect can be expected, the orphan drug funding process ensures that people who experience those disorders can have some hope of pharmacotherapeutic advances.

Targets

The definition of target itself is something argued within the pharmaceutical industry. Generally, the "target" is the naturally existing cellular or molecular structure involved in the pathology of interest that the drug-in-development is meant to act on. However, the distinction between a new and established target can be made without a full understanding of just what a target is. This distinction is typically made by pharmaceutical companies engaged in discovery and development of therapeutics. In an estimate from 2011, 435 human genome products were identified as therapeutic drug targets of FDA-approved drugs.

Established targets are those for which there is a good scientific understanding, supported by a lengthy publication history, of both how the target functions in normal physiology and how it is involved in human pathology. This does not imply that the mechanism of action of drugs that are thought to act through a particular established target is fully understood. Rather, established relates directly to the amount of background information available on a target, in particular functional information. The more such information is available, the less investment is (generally) required to develop a therapeutic directed against the target. The process of gathering such functional information is called "target validation" in pharmaceutical industry parlance. Established targets also include those that the pharmaceutical industry has had experience mounting drug discovery campaigns against in the past; such a history provides information on the chemical feasibility of developing a small molecular therapeutic against the target and can provide licensing opportunities and freedom-to-operate indicators with respect to small-molecule therapeutic candidates.

In general, new targets are all those targets that are not established targets but which have been or are the subject of drug discovery campaigns. These typically include newly discovered proteins, or proteins whose function has now become clear as a result of basic scientific research.

The majority of targets currently selected for drug discovery efforts are proteins. Two classes predominate: G-protein-coupled receptors (or GPCRs) and protein kinases.

Screening and Design

The process of finding a new drug against a chosen target for a particular disease usually involves high-throughput screening (HTS), wherein large libraries of chemicals are tested for their ability to modify the target. For example, if the target is a novel GPCR, compounds will be screened for their ability to inhibit or stimulate that receptor: if the target is a protein kinase, the chemicals will be tested for their ability to inhibit that kinase.

Another important function of HTS is to show how selective the compounds are for the chosen target, as one wants to find a molecule which will interfere with only the chosen target, but not other, related targets. To this end, other screening runs will be made to see whether the hits against the chosen target will interfere with other related targets – this is the process of cross-screening. Cross-screening is important, because the more unrelated targets a compound hits, the more likely that off-target toxicity will occur with that compound once it reaches the clinic.

It is very unlikely that a perfect drug candidate will emerge from these early screening runs. One of the first steps is to screen for compounds that are unlikely to be developed into drugs; for example compounds that are hits in almost every assay, classified by medicinal chemists as "pan-assay interference compounds", are removed at this stage, if they were not already removed from the chemical library. It is often observed that several compounds are found to have some degree of activity, and if these compounds share common chemical features, one or more pharmacophores can then be developed. At this point, medicinal chemists will attempt to use structure-activity relationships (SAR) to improve certain features of the lead compound:

- Increase activity against the chosen target,
- Reduce activity against unrelated targets,
- Improve the druglikeness or ADME properties of the molecule.

This process will require several iterative screening runs, during which, it is hoped, the properties of the new molecular entities will improve, and allow the favoured compounds to go forward to in vitro and in vivo testing for activity in the disease model of choice.

Amongst the physico-chemical properties associated with drug absorption include ionization (pKa), and solubility; permeability can be determined by PAMPA and Caco-2. PAMPA is attractive as an early screen due to the low consumption of drug and the low cost compared to tests such as Caco-2, gastrointestinal tract (GIT) and Blood–brain barrier (BBB) with which there is a high correlation.

A range of parameters can be used to assess the quality of a compound, or a series of compounds, as proposed in the Lipinski's Rule of Five. Such parameters include calculated properties such as cLogP to estimate lipophilicity, molecular weight, polar surface area and measured properties, such as potency, in-vitro measurement of enzymatic clearance etc. Some descriptors such as ligand efficiency (LE) and lipophilic efficiency (LiPE) combine such parameters to assess druglikeness.

While HTS is a commonly used method for novel drug discovery, it is not the only method. It is often possible to start from a molecule which already has some of the desired properties. Such a molecule might be extracted from a natural product or even be a drug on the market which could be improved upon (so-called "me too" drugs). Other methods, such as virtual high throughput screening, where screening is done using computer-generated models and attempting to "dock" virtual libraries to a target, are also often used.

Another important method for drug discovery is de novo drug design, in which a prediction is made of the sorts of chemicals that might (e.g.) fit into an active site of the target enzyme. For example, virtual screening and computer-aided drug design are often used to identify new chemical moieties that may interact with a target protein. Molecular modelling and molecular dynamics simulations can be used as a guide to improve the potency and properties of new drug leads.

There is also a paradigm shift in the drug discovery community to shift away from HTS, which is expensive and may only cover limited chemical space, to the screening of smaller libraries (maximum a few thousand compounds). These include fragment-based lead discovery (FBDD) and protein-directed dynamic combinatorial chemistry. The ligands in these approaches are usually much smaller, and they bind to the target protein with weaker binding affinity than hits that are identified from HTS. Further modifications through organic synthesis into lead compounds are often required. Such modifications are often guided by protein X-ray crystallography of the protein-fragment complex. The advantages of these approaches are that they allow more efficient screening and the compound library, although small, typically covers a large chemical space when compared to HTS.

Phenotypic screens have also provided new chemical starting points in drug discovery. A variety of models have been used including yeast, zebrafish, worms, immortalized cell lines, primary cell lines, patient-derived cell lines and whole animal models. These screens are designed to find compounds which reverse a disease phenotype such as death, protein aggregation, mutant protein expression, or cell proliferation as examples in a more holistic cell model or organism. Smaller screening sets are often used for these screens, especially when the models are expensive or time-consuming to run. In many cases, the exact mechanism of action of hits from these screens is unknown and may require extensive target deconvolution experiments to ascertain.

Once a lead compound series has been established with sufficient target potency and selectivity and favourable drug-like properties, one or two compounds will then be proposed for drug development. The best of these is generally called the lead compound, while the other will be designated as the "backup".

Nature as Source

Traditionally many drugs and other chemicals with biological activity have been discovered by studying allelopathy – chemicals that organisms create that affect the activity of other organisms in the fight for survival.

Despite the rise of combinatorial chemistry as an integral part of lead discovery process, natural products still play a major role as starting material for drug discovery. A 2007 report found that of the 974 small molecule new chemical entities developed between 1981 and 2006, 63% were natural derived or semisynthetic derivatives of natural products. For certain therapy areas, such as antimicrobials, antineoplastics, antihypertensive and anti-inflammatory drugs, the numbers were higher. In many cases, these products have been used traditionally for many years.

Natural products may be useful as a source of novel chemical structures for modern techniques of development of antibacterial therapies.

Despite the implied potential, only a fraction of Earth's living species has been tested for bioactivity.

Plant-derived

Many secondary metabolites produced by plants have potential therapeutic medicinal properties. These secondary metabolites contain bind to and modify the function of proteins (receptors, enzymes, etc.). Consequently, plant derived natural products have often been used as the starting point for drug discovery.

Until the Renaissance, the vast majority of drugs in Western medicine were plant-derived extracts. This has resulted in a pool of information about the potential of plant species as important sources of starting materials for drug discovery. Botanical knowledge about different metabolites and hormones that are produced in different anatomical parts of the plant (e.g. roots, leaves, and flowers) are crucial for correctly identifying bioactive and pharmacological plant properties. Identifying new drugs and getting them approved for market has proved to be a stringent process due to regulations set by national drug regulatory agencies.

Jasmonates

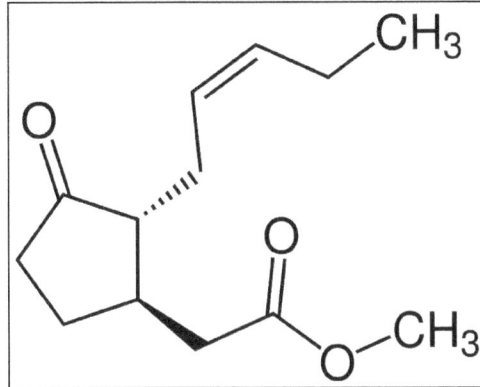

Chemical structure of methyl jasmonate (JA).

Jasmonates are important in responses to injury and intracellular signals. They induce apoptosis and protein cascade via proteinase inhibitor, have defense functions, and regulate plant responses to different biotic and abiotic stresses. Jasmonates also have the ability to directly act on mitochondrial membranes by inducing membrane depolarization via release of metabolites.

Jasmonate derivatives (JAD) are also important in wound response and tissue regeneration in plant cells. They have also been identified to have anti-aging effects on human epidermal layer. It is suspected that interact with proteoglycans (PG) and glycosaminoglycan (GAG) polysaccharides, which are essential extracellular matrix (ECM) components to help remodel the ECM. The discovery of JADs on skin repair has introduced newfound interest in the effects of these plant hormones in therapeutic medicinal application.

Salicylates

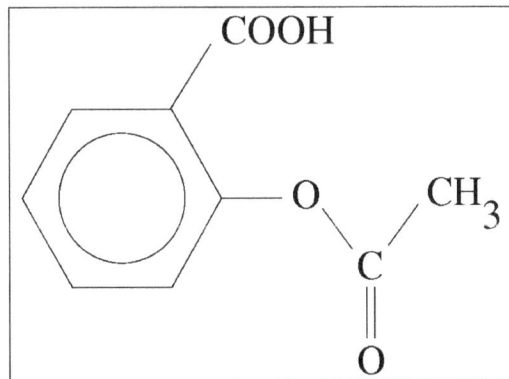

Chemical structure of Acetylsalicylic acid, more commonly known as Aspirin.

Salicylic acid (SA), a phytohormone, was initially derived from willow bark and has since been identified in many species. It is an important player in plant immunity, although its role is still not fully understood by scientists. They are involved in disease and immunity responses in plant and animal tissues. They have salicylic acid binding proteins (SABPs) that have shown to affect multiple animal tissues. The first discovered medicinal properties of the isolated compound was involved in pain and fever management. They also play an active role in the suppression of cell proliferation. They have the ability to induce death in lymphoblastic leukemia and other human cancer cells. One of the most common drugs derived from salicylates is aspirin, also known as acetylsalicylic acid, with anti-inflammatory and anti-pyretic properties.

Microbial Metabolites

Microbes compete for living space and nutrients. To survive in these conditions, many microbes have developed abilities to prevent competing species from proliferating. Microbes are the main source of antimicrobial drugs. Streptomyces isolates have been such a valuable source of antibiotics, that they have been called medicinal molds. The classic example of an antibiotic discovered as a defense mechanism against another microbe is penicillin in bacterial cultures contaminated by *Penicillium* fungi in 1928.

Marine Invertebrates

Marine environments are potential sources for new bioactive agents. Arabinose nucleosides discovered from marine invertebrates in 1950s, demonstrated for the first time that sugar moieties other than ribose and deoxyribose can yield bioactive nucleoside structures. It took until 2004 when the first marine-derived drug was approved. For example, the cone snail toxin ziconotide, also known as Prialt treats severe neuropathic pain. Several other marine-derived agents are now in clinical trials for indications such as cancer, anti-inflammatory use and pain. One class of these agents are bryostatin-like compounds, under investigation as anti-cancer therapy.

Chemical Diversity

Combinatorial chemistry was a key technology enabling the efficient generation of large screening libraries for the needs of high-throughput screening. However, now, after two decades of combinatorial chemistry, it has been pointed out that despite the increased efficiency in chemical synthesis, no increase in lead or drug candidates has been reached. This has led to analysis of chemical characteristics of combinatorial chemistry products, compared to existing drugs or natural products. The chemoinformatics concept chemical diversity, depicted as distribution of compounds in the chemical space based on their physicochemical characteristics, is often used to describe the difference between the combinatorial chemistry libraries and natural products. The synthetic, combinatorial library compounds seem to cover only a limited and quite uniform chemical space, whereas existing drugs and particularly natural products, exhibit much greater chemical diversity, distributing more evenly to the chemical space. The most prominent differences between natural products and compounds in combinatorial chemistry libraries is the number of chiral centers (much higher in natural compounds), structure rigidity (higher in natural compounds) and number of aromatic moieties (higher in combinatorial chemistry libraries). Other chemical differences between these two groups include the nature of heteroatoms (O and N enriched in natural products, and S and halogen atoms more often present in synthetic compounds), as well as level of non-aromatic unsaturation (higher in natural products). As both structure rigidity and chirality are well-established factors in medicinal chemistry known to enhance compounds specificity and efficacy as a drug, it has been suggested that natural products compare favourably to today's combinatorial chemistry libraries as potential lead molecules.

Screening

Two main approaches exist for the finding of new bioactive chemical entities from natural sources.

The first is sometimes referred to as random collection and screening of material, but the collection is far from random. Biological (often botanical) knowledge is often used to identify families that show promise. This approach is effective because only a small part of earth's biodiversity has ever been tested for pharmaceutical activity. Also, organisms living in a species-rich environment need to evolve defensive and competitive mechanisms to survive. Those mechanisms might be exploited in the development of beneficial drugs.

A collection of plant, animal and microbial samples from rich ecosystems can potentially give rise to novel biological activities worth exploiting in the drug development process. One example of a successful use of this strategy is the screening for antitumour agents by the National Cancer Institute, started in the 1960s. Paclitaxel was identified from Pacific yew tree *Taxus brevifolia*. Paclitaxel showed anti-tumour activity by a previously undescribed mechanism (stabilization of microtubules) and is now approved for clinical use for the treatment of lung, breast and ovarian cancer, as well as for Kaposi's sarcoma. Early in the 21st century, Cabazitaxel (made by Sanofi, a French firm), another relative of taxol has been shown effective against prostate cancer, also because it works by preventing the formation of microtubules, which pull the chromosomes apart in dividing cells (such as cancer cells). Other examples are: 1. Camptotheca (Camptothecin, Topotecan, Irinotecan, Rubitecan, Belotecan); 2. Podophyllum (Etoposide, Teniposide); 3a. Anthracyclines (Aclarubicin, Daunorubicin, Doxorubicin, Epirubicin, Idarubicin, Amrubicin, Pirarubicin, Valrubicin, Zorubicin); 3b. Anthracenediones (Mitoxantrone, Pixantrone).

The second main approach involves ethnobotany, the study of the general use of plants in society, and ethnopharmacology, an area inside ethnobotany, which is focused specifically on medicinal uses.

Artemisinin, an antimalarial agent from sweet wormtree *Artemisia annua*, used in Chinese medicine since 200BC is one drug used as part of combination therapy for multiresistant *Plasmodium falciparum*.

Structural Elucidation

The elucidation of the chemical structure is critical to avoid the re-discovery of a chemical agent that is already known for its structure and chemical activity. Mass spectrometry is a method in which individual compounds are identified based on their mass/charge ratio, after ionization. Chemical compounds exist in nature as mixtures, so the combination of liquid chromatography and mass spectrometry (LC-MS) is often used to separate the individual chemicals. Databases of mass spectras for known compounds are available, and can be used to assign a structure to an unknown mass spectrum. Nuclear magnetic resonance spectroscopy is the primary technique for determining chemical structures of natural products. NMR yields information about individual hydrogen and carbon atoms in the structure, allowing detailed reconstruction of the molecule's architecture.

DRUG DEVELOPMENT

Drug development is the process of bringing a new pharmaceutical drug to the market once a lead compound has been identified through the process of drug discovery. It includes preclinical research on microorganisms and animals, filing for regulatory status, such as via the United States Food and Drug Administration for an investigational new drug to initiate clinical trials on humans, and may include the step of obtaining regulatory approval with a new drug application to market the drug.

New Chemical Entity Development

Broadly, the process of drug development can be divided into preclinical and clinical work.

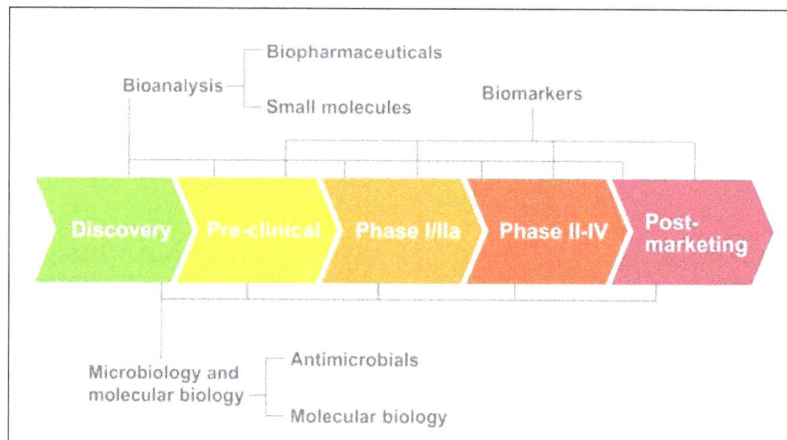

Pre-clinical

New chemical entities (NCEs, also known as new molecular entities or NMEs) are compounds that emerge from the process of drug discovery. These have promising activity against a particular biological target that is important in disease. However, little is known about the safety, toxicity, pharmacokinetics, and metabolism of this NCE in humans. It is the function of drug development to assess all of these parameters prior to human clinical trials. A further major objective of drug development is to recommend the dose and schedule for the first use in a human clinical trial ("first-in-man" [FIM] or First Human Dose [FHD]).

In addition, drug development must establish the physicochemical properties of the NCE: its chemical makeup, stability, and solubility. Manufacturers must optimize the process they use to make the chemical so they can scale up from a medicinal chemist producing milligrams, to manufacturing on the kilogram and ton scale. They further examine the product for suitability to package as capsules, tablets, aerosol, intramuscular injectable, subcutaneous injectable, or intravenous formulations. Together, these processes are known in preclinical and clinical development as chemistry, manufacturing, and control (CMC).

Many aspects of drug development focus on satisfying the regulatory requirements of drug licensing authorities. These generally constitute a number of tests designed to determine the major toxicities of a novel compound prior to first use in humans. It is a legal requirement that an assessment of major organ toxicity be performed (effects on the heart and lungs, brain, kidney, liver and digestive system), as well as effects on other parts of the body that might be affected by the drug (e.g. the skin if the new drug is to be delivered through the skin). Increasingly, these tests are made using *in vitro* methods (e.g. with isolated cells), but many tests can only be made by using experimental animals to demonstrate the complex interplay of metabolism and drug exposure on toxicity.

The information is gathered from this preclinical testing, as well as information on CMC, and submitted to regulatory authorities (in the US, to the FDA), as an Investigational New Drug (IND) application. If the IND is approved, development moves to the clinical phase.

Clinical Phase

Clinical trials involve three or four steps:

- Phase I trials, usually in healthy volunteers, determine safety and dosing.

- Phase II trials are used to get an initial reading of efficacy and further explore safety in small numbers of patients having the disease targeted by the NCE.

- Phase III trials are large, pivotal trials to determine safety and efficacy in sufficiently large numbers of patients with the targeted disease. If safety and efficacy are adequately proved, clinical testing may stop at this step and the NCE advances to the new drug application (NDA) stage.

- Phase IV trials are post-approval trials that are sometimes a condition attached by the FDA, also called post-market surveillance studies.

The process of defining characteristics of the drug does not stop once an NCE begins human clinical trials. In addition to the tests required to move a novel drug into the clinic for the first time, manufacturers must ensure that any long-term or chronic toxicities are well-defined, including effects on systems not previously monitored (fertility, reproduction, immune system, among others). They must also test the compound for its potential to cause cancer (carcinogenicity testing).

If a compound emerges from these tests with an acceptable toxicity and safety profile, and the company can further show it has the desired effect in clinical trials, then the NCE portfolio of evidence can be submitted for marketing approval in the various countries where the manufacturer plans to sell it. In the United States, this process is called a "new drug application" or NDA.

Most NCEs fail during drug development, either because they have unacceptable toxicity or because they simply do not have the intended effect on the targeted disease as shown in clinical trials.

A trend toward the collection of biomarker and genetic information from clinical trial participants, and increasing investment by companies in this area, led by 2018 to fully half of all drug trials collecting this information, the prevalence reaching above 80% among oncology trials.

Cost

The full cost of bringing a new drug (i.e. new chemical entity) to market – from discovery through clinical trials to approval – is complex and controversial. Typically, companies spend tens to hundreds of millions of U.S. dollars. One element of the complexity is that the much-publicized final numbers often not only include the out-of-pocket expenses for conducting a series of Phase I-III clinical trials, but also the capital costs of the long period (10 or more years) during which the company must cover out-of-pocket costs for preclinical drug discovery. Additionally, companies often do not report whether a given figure includes the capitalized cost or comprises only out-of-pocket expenses, or both. Another element of complexity is that all estimates are based on voluntary releases of otherwise confidential information which may not be easily independently verified.

One 2010 study assessed both capitalized and out-of-pocket costs for bringing a single new drug to market as about US$1.8 billion and $870 million, respectively.

In an analysis of the drug development costs for 98 companies over a decade, the average cost per drug developed and approved by a single-drug company was $350 million. But for companies that approved between eight and 13 drugs over 10 years, the cost per drug went as high as $5.5 billion, due mainly to geographic expansion for marketing and ongoing costs for Phase IV trials and continuous monitoring for safety.

Alternatives to conventional drug development have the objective for universities, governments, and the pharmaceutical industry to collaborate and optimize resources.

Valuation

The nature of a drug development project is characterised by high attrition rates, large capital expenditures, and long timelines. This makes the valuation of such projects and companies a challenging task. Not all valuation methods can cope with these particularities. The most commonly used valuation methods are risk-adjusted net present value (rNPV), decision trees, real options, or comparables.

The most important value drivers are the cost of capital or discount rate that is used, phase attributes such as duration, success rates, and costs, and the forecasted sales, including cost of goods and marketing and sales expenses. Less objective aspects like quality of the management or novelty of the technology should be reflected in the cash flows estimation.

Success Rate

Candidates for a new drug to treat a disease might, theoretically, include from 5,000 to 10,000 chemical compounds. On average about 250 of these show sufficient promise for further evaluation using laboratory tests, mice and other test animals. Typically, about ten of these qualify for tests on humans. A study conducted by the Tufts Center for the Study of Drug Development covering the 1980s and 1990s found that only 21.5 percent of drugs that started Phase I trials were eventually approved for marketing. In the time period of 2006 to 2015, the success rate was 9.6%. The high failure rates associated with pharmaceutical development are referred to as the "attrition rate" problem. Careful decision making during drug development is essential to avoid costly failures. In many cases, intelligent programme and clinical trial design can prevent false negative results. Well-designed, dose-finding studies and comparisons against both a placebo and a gold-standard treatment arm play a major role in achieving reliable data.

Novel Initiatives to Boost Development

Novel initiatives include partnering between governmental organizations and industry. The world's largest such initiative is the Innovative Medicines Initiative (IMI), and examples of major national initiatives are Top Institute Pharma in the Netherlands and Biopeople in Denmark. In 2004, the FDA created the "Critical Path Initiative" to guide the new drug development process. In 2012, the Food and Drug Administration Safety and Innovation Act created the breakthrough therapy designation.

DRUG DELIVERY

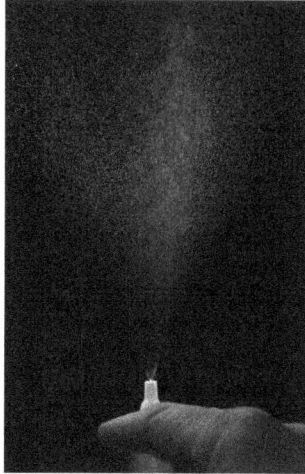

A nasal spray bottle being demonstrated.

Drug delivery refers to approaches, formulations, technologies, and systems for transporting a pharmaceutical compound in the body as needed to safely achieve its desired therapeutic effect. It may involve scientific site-targeting within the body, or it might involve facilitating systemic pharmacokinetics; in any case, it is typically concerned with both quantity and duration of drug presence. Drug delivery is often approached via a drug's chemical formulation, but it may also involve medical devices or drug-device combination products. Drug delivery is a concept heavily integrated with dosage form and route of administration, the latter sometimes even being considered part of the definition.

Drug delivery technologies modify drug release profile, absorption, distribution and elimination for the benefit of improving product efficacy and safety, as well as patient convenience and compliance. Drug release is from: diffusion, degradation, swelling, and affinity-based mechanisms. Some of the common routes of administration include the enteral (gastrointestinal tract), parenteral (via injections), inhalation, transdermal, topical and oral routes. Many medications such as peptide and protein, antibody, vaccine and gene based drugs, in general may not be delivered using these routes because they might be susceptible to enzymatic degradation or can not be absorbed into the systemic circulation efficiently due to molecular size and charge issues to be therapeutically effective. For this reason many protein and peptide drugs have to be delivered by injection or a nanoneedle array. For example, many immunizations are based on the delivery of protein drugs and are often done by injection.

Current efforts in the area of drug delivery include the development of targeted delivery in which the drug is only active in the target area of the body (for example, in cancerous tissues), sustained release formulations in which the drug is released over a period of time in a controlled manner from a formulation, and methods to increase survival of peroral agents which must pass through the stomach's acidic environment. In order to achieve efficient targeted delivery, the designed system must avoid the host's defense mechanisms and circulate to its intended site of action. Types of sustained release formulations include liposomes, drug loaded biodegradable microspheres and drug polymer conjugates. Survival of agents as they pass through the stomach typically is an issue for agents which cannot be encased in a solid tablet; one research area has been around the utilization of lipid isolates from the acid-resistant archaea *Sulfolobus islandicus*, which confers on the order of 10% survival of liposome-encapsulated agents.

DRUG DETOXIFICATION

Drug detoxification is variously the intervention in a case of physical dependence to a drug; the process and experience of a withdrawal syndrome; and any of various treatments for acute drug overdose.

A detoxification program for physical dependence does not necessarily address the precedents of addiction, social factors, psychological addiction, or the often-complex behavioral issues that intermingle with addiction.

The United States Department of Health and Human Services acknowledges three steps in a drug detoxification process:

1. Evaluation: Upon beginning drug detoxification, a patient is first tested to see which specific substances are presently circulating in their bloodstream and the amount. Clinicians also evaluate the patient for potential co-occurring disorders, dual diagnosis, and mental/behavioral issues.

2. Stabilization: In this stage, the patient is guided through the process of detoxification. This may be done with or without the use of medications but for the most part the former is more common. Also part of stabilization is explaining to the patient what to expect during treatment and the recovery process. Where appropriate, people close to the addict are brought in at this time to become involved and show support.

3. Guiding Patient into Treatment: The last step of the detoxification process is to ready the patient for the actual recovery process. As drug detoxification only deals with the physical dependency and addiction to drugs, it does not address

the psychological aspects of drug addiction. This stage entails obtaining agreement from the patient to complete the process by enrolling in a drug rehabilitation program.

Rapid Detoxification

The principle of rapid detoxification is to use heavy sedation alongside dosing with opioid antagonists. This approach is expensive, ineffective and extremely dangerous.

LIFESTYLE DRUG

Lifestyle drug is an imprecise term commonly applied to medications which treat non–life-threatening and non-painful conditions such as baldness, wrinkles, erectile dysfunction, or acne, which the speaker perceives as either not medical problems at all or as minor medical conditions relative to others. It is sometimes intended as a pejorative, bearing the implication that the scarce medical research resources allocated to develop such drugs were spent frivolously when they could have been better spent researching cures for more serious medical conditions. Proponents, however, point out that improving the patient's subjective quality of life has always been a primary concern of medicine, and argue that these drugs are doing just that. It finds broad use in both media and scholarly journals.

Concept and Impact on Society

There is direct impact of lifestyle drugs on society, particularly in the developing world. Implications associated with labeling of indications and products sales of these lifestyle drugs may be varied. Drugs can, over time, switch from 'lifestyle' to 'mainstream' use.

Bioethics and Medical Policy Debate

Though no precise widely accepted definition or criteria are associated with the term, there is much debate within the fields of pharmacology and bioethics around the propriety of developing such drugs, particularly after the commercial debut of Viagra.

Critics of pharmaceutical firms claim that pharmaceutical firms actively medicalize; that is, they invent novel disorders and diseases which were not recognized as such before their "cures" could be profitably marketed, in effect pathologizing what were widely regarded as normal conditions of human existence. The consequences are said to include generally greater worries about health, misallocation of limited medical research resources to comparatively minor conditions while many serious diseases remain uncured, and needless health care expenditure. This medicalization of some element of human condition has significance, in principle, as a matter for political discourse or dialogue in civil society concerning values or morals.

Social critics also question the propriety of devoting huge research budgets towards creating these drugs when far more dangerous diseases like cancer and AIDS remain uncured. It is sometimes claimed that lifestyle drugs amount to little more than medically sanctioned recreational drug use.

DRUG INTERACTION

A drug interaction is a change in the action or side effects of a drug caused by concomitant administration with a food, beverage, supplement, or another drug.

There are many causes of drug interactions. For example, one drug may alter the pharmacokinetics of another. Alternatively, drug interactions may result from competition for a single receptor or signaling pathway.

The risk of a drug-drug interaction increases with the number of drugs used. Over a third (36%) of the elderly in the U.S. regularly use five or more medications or supplements, and 15% are at risk of a significant drug-drug interaction.

Pharmacodynamic Interactions

When two drugs are used together, their effects can be additive (the result is what you expect when you add together the effect of each drug taken independently), synergistic (combining the drugs leads to a larger effect than expected), or antagonistic (combining the drugs leads to a smaller effect than expected). There is sometimes confusion on whether drugs are synergistic or additive, since the individual effects of each drug may vary from patient to patient. A synergistic interaction may be beneficial for patients, but may also increase the risk of overdose.

Both synergy and antagonism can occur during different phases of the interaction between a drug, and an organism. For example, when synergy occurs at a cellular receptor level this is termed agonism, and the substances involved are termed agonists. On the other hand, in the case of antagonism, the substances involved are known as inverse agonists. The different responses of a receptor to the action of a drug has resulted in a number of classifications, such as "partial agonist", "competitive agonist" etc. These concepts have fundamental applications in the pharmacodynamics of these interactions. The proliferation of existing classifications at this level, along with the fact that the exact reaction mechanisms for many drugs are not well-understood means that it is almost impossible to offer a clear classification for these concepts. It is even possible that many authors would misapply any given classification.

Direct interactions between drugs are also possible and may occur when two drugs are mixed prior to intravenous injection. For example, mixing thiopentone and suxamethonium in the same syringe can lead to the precipitation of thiopentone.

The change in an organism's response upon administration of a drug is an important factor in pharmacodynamic interactions. These changes are extraordinarily difficult to classify given the wide variety of modes of action that exist, and the fact that many drugs can cause their effect through a number of different mechanisms. This wide diversity also means that, in all but the most obvious cases it is important to investigate, and understand these mechanisms. The well-founded suspicion exists that there are more unknown interactions than known ones.

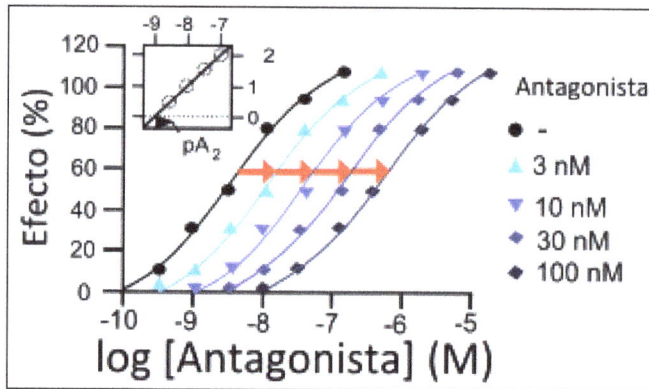

Effects of the competitive inhibition of an agonist by increases in the concentration of an antagonist. A drugs potency can be affected (the response curve shifted to the right) by the presence of an antagonistic interaction. pA_2 known as the Schild representation, a mathematical model of the agonist: antagonist relationship or vice versa. NB: the x-axis is incorrectly labelled and should reflect the agonist concentration, not antagonist concentration.

Pharmacodynamic interactions can occur on:

1. Pharmacological receptors: Receptor interactions are the most easily defined, but they are also the most common. From a pharmacodynamic perspective, two drugs can be considered to be:

   - Homodynamic, if they act on the same receptor. They, in turn can be:

     ○ Pure agonists, if they bind to the main locus of the receptor, causing a similar effect to that of the main drug.

     ○ Partial agonists if, on binding to one of the receptor's secondary sites, they have the same effect as the main drug, but with a lower intensity.

     ○ Antagonists, if they bind directly to the receptor's main locus but their effect is opposite to that of the main drug. These include:

       ▪ Competitive antagonists, if they compete with the main drug to bind with the receptor. The amount of antagonist or main drug that binds with the receptor will depend on the concentrations of each one in the plasma.

- Uncompetitive antagonists, when the antagonist binds to the receptor irreversibly and is not released until the receptor is saturated. In principle the quantity of antagonist and agonist that binds to the receptor will depend on their concentrations. However, the presence of the antagonist will cause the main drug to be released from the receptor regardless of the main drug's concentration, therefore all the receptors will eventually become occupied by the antagonist.

- Heterodynamic competitors, if they act on distinct receptors.

2. Signal transduction mechanisms: These are molecular processes that commence after the interaction of the drug with the receptor. For example, it is known that hypoglycaemia (low blood glucose) in an organism produces a release of catecholamines, which trigger compensation mechanisms thereby increasing blood glucose levels. The release of catecholamines also triggers a series of symptoms, which allows the organism to recognise what is happening and which act as a stimulant for preventative action (eating sugars). Should a patient be taking a drug such as insulin, which reduces glycaemia, and also be taking another drug such as certain beta-blockers for heart disease, then the beta-blockers will act to block the adrenaline receptors. This will block the reaction triggered by the catecholamines should a hypoglycaemic episode occur. Therefore, the body will not adopt corrective mechanisms and there will be an increased risk of a serious reaction resulting from the ingestion of both drugs at the same time.

3. Antagonic physiological systems: Imagine a drug A that acts on a certain organ. This effect will increase with increasing concentrations of physiological substance S in the organism. Now imagine a drug B that acts on another organ, which increases the amount of substance S. If both drugs are taken simultaneously it is possible that drug A could cause an adverse reaction in the organism as its effect will be indirectly increased by the action of drug B. An actual example of this interaction is found in the concomitant use of digoxin and furosemide. The former acts on cardiac fibres and its effect is increased if there are low levels of potassium (K) in blood plasma. Furosemide is a diuretic that lowers arterial tension but favours the loss of K^+. This could lead to hypokalemia (low levels of potassium in the blood), which could increase the toxicity of digoxin.

Pharmacokinetic Interactions

Modifications in the effect of a drug are caused by differences in the absorption, transport, distribution, metabolism or excretion of one or both of the drugs compared with the expected behavior of each drug when taken individually. These changes are basically modifications in the concentration of the drugs. In this respect, two drugs can be homergic if they have the same effect in the organism and heterergic if their effects are different.

Absorption Interactions

Changes in Motility

Some drugs, such as the prokinetic agents increase the speed with which a substance passes through the intestines. If a drug is present in the digestive tract's absorption zone for less time its blood concentration will decrease. The opposite will occur with drugs that decrease intestinal motility.

- pH: Drugs can be present in either ionised or non-ionised form, depending on their pKa (pH at which the drug reaches equilibrium between its ionised and non-ionised form). The non-ionized forms of drugs are usually easier to absorb, because they will not be repelled by the lipidic bylayer of the cell, most of them can be absorbed by passive diffusion, unless they are too big or too polarized (like glucose or vancomycin), in which case they may have or not have specific and non specific transporters distributed on the entire intestine internal surface, that carries drugs inside the body. Obviously increasing the absorption of a drug will increase its bioavailability, so, changing the drug's state between ionized or not, can be useful or not for certain drugs.

  Certain drugs require an acid stomach pH for absorption. Others require the basic pH of the intestines. Any modification in the pH could change this absorption. In the case of the antacids, an increase in pH can inhibit the absorption of other drugs such as zalcitabine (absorption can be decreased by 25%), tipranavir (25%) and amprenavir (up to 35%). However, this occurs less often than an increase in pH causes an increase in absorption. Such as occurs when cimetidine is taken with didanosine. In this case a gap of two to four hours between taking the two drugs is usually sufficient to avoid the interaction.

- Drug solubility: The absorption of some drugs can be drastically reduced if they are administered together with food with a high fat content. This is the case for oral anticoagulants and avocado.

- Formation of non-absorbable complexes:

  ○ Chelation: The presence of di- or trivalent cations can cause the chelation of certain drugs, making them harder to absorb. This interaction frequently occurs between drugs such as tetracycline or the fluoroquinolones and dairy products (due to the presence of Ca^{++}).

- ◦ Binding with proteins: Some drugs such as sucralfate binds to proteins, especially if they have a high bioavailability. For this reason its administration is contraindicated in enteral feeding.

- ◦ Finally, another possibility is that the drug is retained in the intestinal lumen forming large complexes that impede its absorption. This can occur with cholestyramine if it is associated with sulfamethoxazol, thyroxine, warfarin or digoxin.

- Acting on the P-glycoprotein of the enterocytes: This appears to be one of the mechanisms promoted by the consumption of grapefruit juice in increasing the bioavailability of various drugs, regardless of its demonstrated inhibitory activity on first pass metabolism.

Transport and Distribution Interactions

The main interaction mechanism is competition for plasma protein transport. In these cases the drug that arrives first binds with the plasma protein, leaving the other drug dissolved in the plasma, which modifies its concentration. The organism has mechanisms to counteract these situations (by, for example, increasing plasma clearance), which means that they are not usually clinically relevant. However, these situations should be taken into account if other associated problems are present such as when the method of excretion is affected.

Metabolism Interactions

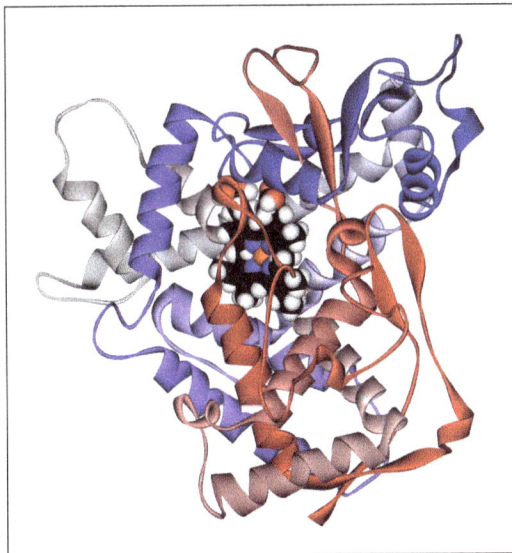

Diagram of cytochrome P450 isoenzyme 2C9 with the haem group in the centre of the enzyme.

Many drug interactions are due to alterations in drug metabolism. Further, human drug-metabolizing enzymes are typically activated through the engagement of nuclear receptors. One notable system involved in metabolic drug interactions is the enzyme system comprising the cytochrome P450 oxidases.

CYP450

Cytochrome P450 is a very large family of haemoproteins (hemoproteins) that are characterized by their enzymatic activity and their role in the metabolism of a large number of drugs. Of the various families that are present in human beings the most interesting in this respect are the 1, 2 and 3, and the most important enzymes are CYP1A2, CYP2C9, CYP2C19, CYP2D6, CYP2E1 and CYP3A4. The majority of the enzymes are also involved in the metabolism of endogenous substances, such as steroids or sex hormones, which is also important should there be interference with these substances. As a result of these interactions the function of the enzymes can either be stimulated (enzyme induction) or inhibited (enzyme inhibition).

Enzymatic Inhibition

If drug A is metabolized by a cytochrome P450 enzyme and drug B inhibits or decreases the enzyme's activity, then drug A will remain with high levels in the plasma for longer as its inactivation is slower. As a result, enzymatic inhibition will cause an increase in the drug's effect. This can cause a wide range of adverse reactions.

It is possible that this can occasionally lead to a paradoxical situation, where the enzymatic inhibition causes a decrease in the drug's effect: if the metabolism of drug A gives rise to product A_2, which actually produces the effect of the drug. If the metabolism of drug A is inhibited by drug B the concentration of A_2 that is present in the blood will decrease, as will the final effect of the drug.

Enzymatic Induction

If drug A is metabolized by a cytochrome P450 enzyme and drug B induces or increases the enzyme's activity, then blood plasma concentrations of drug A will quickly fall as its inactivation will take place more rapidly. As a result, enzymatic induction will cause a decrease in the drug's effect.

As in the previous case, it is possible to find paradoxical situations where an active metabolite causes the drug's effect. In this case the increase in active metabolite A_2 (following the previous example) produces an increase in the drug's effect.

It can often occur that a patient is taking two drugs that are enzymatic inductors, one inductor and the other inhibitor or both inhibitors, which greatly complicates the control of an individual's medication and the avoidance of possible adverse reactions.

An example of this is shown in the following table for the CYP1A2 enzyme, which is the most common enzyme found in the human liver. The table shows the substrates (drugs metabolized by this enzyme) and the inductors and inhibitors of its activity:

Drugs related to CYP1A2		
Substrates	Inhibitors	Inductors
• Caffeine	• Omeprazole	• Phenobarbital
• Theophylline	• Nicotine	• Fluvoxamine
• Phenacetin	• Cimetidine	• Venlafaxine
• Clomipramine	• Ciprofloxacin	• Ticlopidine
• Clozapine		
• Thioridazine		

Enzyme CYP3A4 is the enzyme that the greatest number of drugs use as a substrate. Over 100 drugs depend on its metabolism for their activity and many others act on the enzyme as inductors or inhibitors.

Some foods also act as inductors or inhibitors of enzymatic activity.

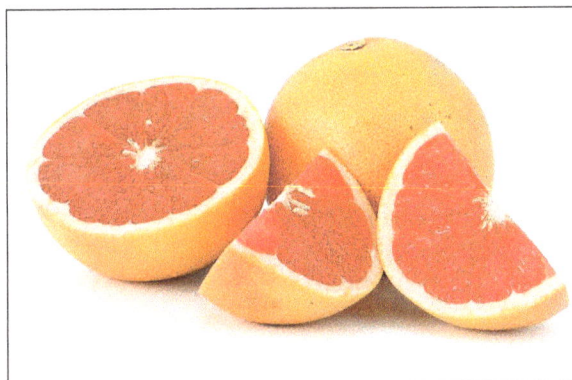

Grapefruit juice can act as an enzyme inhibitor.

Any study of pharmacological interactions between particular medicines should also discuss the likely interactions of some medicinal plants. The effects caused by medicinal plants should be considered in the same way as those of medicines as their interaction with the organism gives rise to a pharmacological response. Other drugs can modify this response and also the plants can give rise to changes in the effects of other active ingredients.

There is little data available regarding interactions involving medicinal plants for the following reasons:

1. False sense of security regarding medicinal plants. The interaction between a medicinal plant and a drug is usually overlooked due to a belief in the "safety of medicinal plants."

2. Variability of composition, both qualitative and quantitative. The composition of a plant-based drug is often subject to wide variations due to a number of factors such as seasonal differences in concentrations, soil type, climatic changes or the existence of different varieties or chemical races within the same plant species that have variable compositions of the active ingredient. On occasion, an interaction can be due to just one active ingredient, but this can be absent in some chemical varieties or it can be present in low concentrations, which will not cause an interaction. Counter interactions can even occur. This occurs, for instance, with ginseng, the *Panax ginseng* variety increases the Prothrombin time, while the *Panax quinquefolius* variety decreases it.

3. Absence of use in at-risk groups, such as hospitalized and polypharmacy patients, who tend to have the majority of drug interactions.

4. Limited consumption of medicinal plants has given rise to a lack of interest in this area.

They are usually included in the category of foods as they are usually taken as a tea or food supplement. However, medicinal plants are increasingly being taken in a manner more often associated with conventional medicines: pills, tablets, capsules, etc.

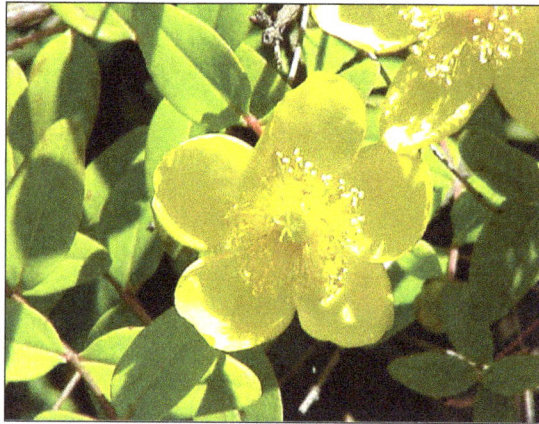

St John's wort can act as an enzyme inductor.

Excretion Interactions

Renal Excretion

Only the free fraction of a drug that is dissolved in the blood plasma can be removed through the kidney. Therefore, drugs that are tightly bound to proteins are not available for renal excretion, as long as they are not metabolized when they may be eliminated as metabolites. Creatinine clearance is used as a measure of kidney functioning but it is only useful in cases where the drug is excreted in an unaltered form in the urine. The excretion of drugs from the kidney's nephrons has the same properties as that of any other organic solute: Passive filtration, reabsorption and active secretion. In the latter phase the secretion of drugs is an active process that is subject to conditions relating to the saturability of the transported molecule and competition between substrates. Therefore, these are key sites where interactions between drugs could occur.

Filtration depends on a number of factors including the pH of the urine, it having been shown that the drugs that act as weak bases are increasingly excreted as the pH of the urine becomes more acidic, and the inverse is true for weak acids. This mechanism is of great use when treating intoxications (by making the urine more acidic or more alkali) and it is also used by some drugs and herbal products to produce their interactive effect.

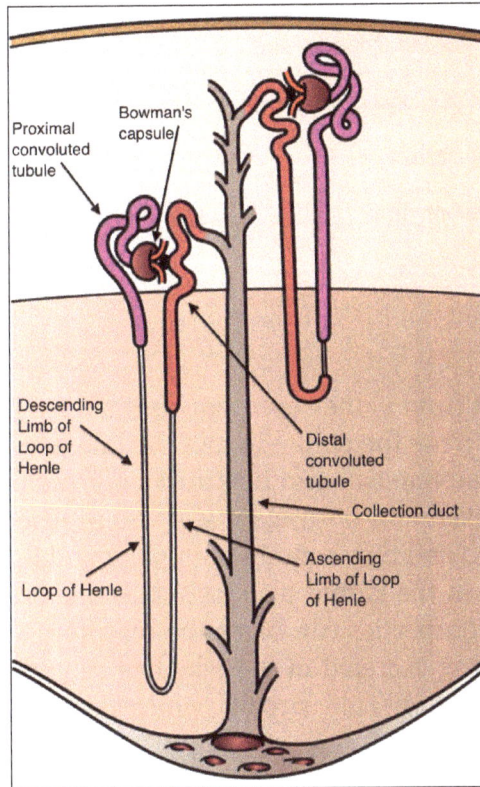

Human kidney nephron.

Drugs that act as weak acids or bases	
Weak acids	Weak bases
• Acetylsalicylic acid	• Reserpine
• Furosemide	• Amphetamine
• Ibuprofen	• Procaine
• Levodopa	• Ephedrine
• Acetazolamide	• Atropine

• Sulfadiazine	• Diazepam
• Ampicillin	• Hydralazine
• Chlorothiazide	• Pindolol
• Paracetamol	• Propranolol
• Chloropropamide	• Salbutamol
• Cromoglicic acid	• Alprenolol
• Ethacrynic acid	• Terbutaline
• alpha-Methyldopamine	• Amiloride
• Phenobarbital	• Chlorpheniramine
• Warfarin	
• Theophylline	
• Phenytoin	

Bile Excretion

Bile excretion is different from kidney excretion as it always involves energy expenditure in active transport across the epithelium of the bile duct against a concentration gradient. This transport system can also be saturated if the plasma concentrations of the drug are high. Bile excretion of drugs mainly takes place where their molecular weight is greater than 300 and they contain both polar and lipophilic groups. The glucuronidation of the drug in the kidney also facilitates bile excretion. Substances with similar physicochemical properties can block the receptor, which is important in assessing interactions. A drug excreted in the bile duct can occasionally be reabsorbed by the intestines (in the enterohepatic circuit), which can also lead to interactions with other drugs.

Herb-drug Interactions

Herb-drug interactions are drug interactions that occur between herbal medicines and conventional drugs. These types of interactions may be more common than drug-drug interactions because herbal medicines often contain multiple pharmacologically active ingredients, while conventional drugs typically contain only one. Some such interactions are clinically significant, although most herbal remedies are not associated with drug interactions causing serious consequences. Most herb-drug interactions are moderate in severity. The most commonly implicated conventional drugs in herb-drug interactions are warfarin, insulin, aspirin, digoxin, and ticlopidine, due to their narrow therapeutic indices. The most commonly implicated herbs involved in such interactions are those containing St. John's Wort, magnesium, calcium, iron, or ginkgo.

Examples of herb-drug interactions include, but are not limited to:

- St. John's wort affects the clearance of numerous drugs, including cyclosporin, SSRI antidepressants, digoxin, indinavir, and phenprocoumon. It may also interact with the anti-cancer drugs irinotecan and imatinib.

- Salvia miltiorrhiza may enhance anticoagulation and bleeding among people taking warfarin.

- Allium sativum has been found to decrease the plasma concentration of saquinavir, and may cause hypoglycemia when taken with chlorpropamide.

- Ginkgo biloba can cause bleeding when combined with warfarin or aspirin.

- Concomitant ephedra and caffeine use has been reported to, in rare cases, cause fatalities.

Mechanisms

The mechanisms underlying most herb-drug interactions are not fully understood. Interactions between herbal medicines and anticancer drugs typically involve enzymes that metabolize cytochrome P450. For example, St. John's Wort has been shown to induce CYP3A4 and P-glycoprotein in vitro and in vivo.

Underlying Factors

It is possible to take advantage of positive drug interactions. However, the negative interactions are usually of more interest because of their pathological significance, and also because they are often unexpected, and may even go undiagnosed. By studying the conditions that favor the appearance of interactions, it should be possible to prevent them, or at least diagnose them in time. The factors or conditions that predispose the appearance of interactions include:

- Old age: Factors relating to how human physiology changes with age may affect the interaction of drugs. For example, liver metabolism, kidney function, nerve transmission or the functioning of bone marrow all decrease with age. In addition, in old age there is a sensory decrease that increases the chances of errors being made in the administration of drugs.

- Polypharmacy: The use of multiple drugs by a single patient, to treat one or more ailments. The more drugs a patient takes the more likely it will be that some of them will interact.

- Genetic factors: Genes synthesize enzymes that metabolize drugs. Some races have genotypic variations that could decrease or increase the activity of these enzymes. The consequence of this would, on occasions, be a greater predisposition towards drug interactions and therefore a greater predisposition for adverse effects to occur. This is seen in genotype variations in the isozymes of cytochrome P450.

- Hepatic or renal diseases: The blood concentrations of drugs that are metabolized in the liver and/or eliminated by the kidneys may be altered if either of these organs is not functioning correctly. If this is the case an increase in blood concentration is normally seen.

- Serious diseases that could worsen if the dose of the medicine is reduced.

- Drug dependent factors:

  ○ Narrow therapeutic index: Where the difference between the effective dose and the toxic dose is small. The drug digoxin is an example of this type of drug.

  ○ Steep dose-response curve: Small changes in the dosage of a drug produce large changes in the drug's concentration in the patient's blood plasma.

  ○ Saturable hepatic metabolism: In addition to dose effects the capacity to metabolize the drug is greatly decreased.

Epidemiology

Among US adults older than 55, 4% are taking medication and or supplements that put them at risk of a major drug interaction. Potential drug-drug interactions have increased over time and are more common in the low educated elderly even after controlling for age, sex, place of residence, and comorbidity.

PRESCRIPTION DRUG

Prescription drugs are often strong medications, which is why they require a prescription from a doctor or dentist. There are three kinds of prescription drugs that are commonly misused:

- Opioids—Used to relieve pain, such as Vicodin, OxyContin, or codeine.

- Depressants—Used to relieve anxiety or help a person sleep, such as Valium or Xanax.

- Stimulants— Used for treating attention deficit hyperactivity disorder (ADHD), such as Adderall and Ritalin.

Prescription drug misuse has become a large public health problem, because misuse can lead to addiction, and even overdose deaths.

What makes Prescription Drugs Unsafe?

Every medication has some risk for harmful effects, sometimes serious ones. Doctors and dentists consider the potential benefits and risks to each patient before prescribing medications and take into account a lot of different factors, described below. When prescription drugs are misused, they can be just as dangerous as drugs that are made illegally.

- Personal information: Before prescribing a drug, health providers consider a person's weight, how long they've been prescribed the medication, other medical conditions, and what other medications they are taking. Someone misusing prescription drugs may overload their system or put themselves at risk for dangerous drug interactions that can cause seizures, coma, or even death.

- Form and dose: Doctors know how long it takes for a pill or capsule to dissolve in the stomach, release drugs to the blood, and reach the brain. When misused, prescription drugs are sometimes taken in larger amounts or in ways that change the way the drug works in the body and brain, putting the person at greater risk for an overdose. For example, when people who misuse OxyContin crush and inhale the pills, a dose that normally works over the course of 12 hours hits the central nervous system all at once. This effect increases the risk for addiction and overdose.

- Side effects: Prescription drugs are designed to treat a specific illness or condition, but they often affect the body in other ways, some of which can be uncomfortable, and in some cases, dangerous. These are called side effects. Side effects can be worse when prescription drugs are not taken as prescribed or are used in combination with other substances.

How Prescription Drugs are Misused?

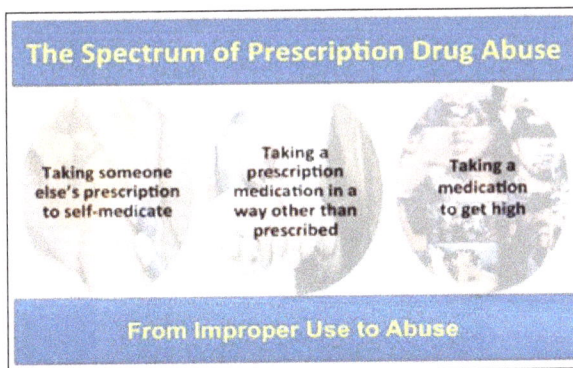

The Spectrum of Prescription Drug Abuse

Taking someone else's prescription to self-medicate

Taking a prescription medication in a way other than prescribed

Taking a medication to get high

From Improper Use to Abuse

- Taking someone else's prescription medication, even if it is for a medical reason (such as to relieve pain, to stay awake, or to fall asleep).

- Taking a prescription medication in a way other than prescribed—for instance, taking more than the prescribed dose or taking it more often, or crushing pills into powder to snort or inject the drug.

- Taking your own prescription in a way that it is not meant to be taken is also misuse. This includes taking more of the medication than prescribed or changing its form—for example, breaking or crushing a pill or capsule and then snorting the powder.

- Taking the prescription medication to get "high."

- Mixing it with alcohol or certain other drugs. Your pharmacist can tell you what other drugs are safe to use with specific prescription drugs.

ROUTES OF DRUG ADMINISTRATION

The path taken by the drug to get into the body is known as the route of drug administration. A drug may be in ionized or unionized form.

Classification

- Enteral route,

- Parenteral route,

- Inhalation,

- Topical.

Enteral Route

Enteral route is through the alimentary canal. It might be:

- Oral,

- Sublingual,

- Per rectum.

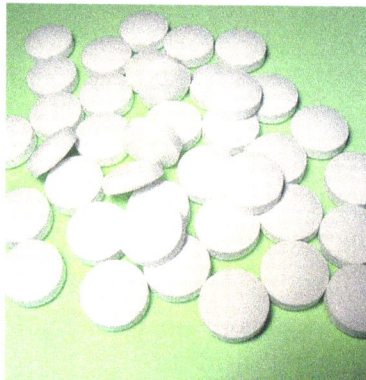

Oral Route

Oral route is the most common route of drug administration. It is mostly used for the neutral drugs. It may be in the form of tablets, capsules, syrup, emulsions or powders.

Advantages

1. It is convenient.

2. It is the cheapest available route.

3. It is easy to use.

4. It is safe and acceptable.

Disadvantages

1. Less amount of drug reaches the target tissue.

2. Some of the drug is destroyed by gastric juices e.g. adrenaline, insulin, oxytocin.

3. Absorption has to take place which is slow, so is not preferred during emergency.

4. It might cause gastric irritation.

5. It might be objectionable in taste.

6. It might cause discoloration of teeth e.g. iron causes staining, tetracyclines below 14 cause brown discoloration so are not advisable during pregnancy.

First Pass Effect

First pass effect is the term used for hepatic metabolism of drug when absorbed and delivered through portal blood. Greater the first pass effect, less amounts of the drug reach the systemic circulation.

Sublingual Route

Sublingual route involves tablets placed under the tongue or between cheeks or Gingiva. The drug should be lipid soluble and small.

Advantages

1. Rapid absorption takes place.

2. Drug is dissolved easily.

3. Drug enters the blood directly.

4. Less first pass effect.

5. Spitting out of the drug removes its effect.

Disadvantages

1. This method is inconvenient.

2. Irritation of the mucous membrane might occur.

3. Person may swallow the drug.

4. Might be unpleasant in taste.

Examples of drugs given by this route include nitroglycerin, isoprenaline and oxytocin. Nifedipine used for the treatment of hypertension in emergency is given by sublingual route.

Rectal Route

Drugs in solid forms such as suppositories or in liquid forms such as enema are given by this route. This route is mostly used in old patients. Drugs may have local or systemic actions after absorption.

Advantages

1. This route is preferred in unconscious or uncooperative patients.

2. This route avoids nausea or vomiting.

3. Drug cannot be destroyed by enzymes.

4. This route is preferred if drug is irritant.

Disadvantages

1. This route is generally not acceptable by the patients.

2. Locally acting drugs include glycerin and Bisacodyl suppository.

3. Systemic acting drugs include Indomethacin (anti inflammatory) and aminophyllin (bronchodilator).

4. Retention enema is diagnostic and is used for finding the pathology of lower intestines.

5. Drugs given by rectal route have 50% first pass metabolism.

Parenteral Route

Injections

1. Intra muscular,

2. Intra venous,

3. Intra-arterial,

4. Intra-cardiac,

5. Intra-thecal,

6. Intraosseous- into bone marrow,

7. Intrapleural,

8. Intraperitoneal,

9. Intra-articular,

10. Intradermal (Intracutaneous),

11. Subcutaneous route (Hypodermic).

Inhalation:Hypospray or Jet Injections.

Advantages

1. Parenteral route is rapid,

2. It is useful for uncooperative patients,

3. It is useful for unconscious patients,

4. Inactivation by GIT enzymes is avoided,

5. First pass effect is avoided,

6. Bioavailability is 100%.

Disadvantages

1. Skill is required,

2. It is painful,

3. This method is expensive,

4. It is less safe.

Classification

Site of Release

Site of release may be intradermal, intraperitoneal, intrapleural, intracardiac, intra-arterial, intrathecal (into meninges of spinal cord), intra-articular (into joint cavity).

Subcutaneous: Subcutaneous route might be used for the arm, forearm, thigh and subscapular space. The volume used is 2 ml. Insoluble suspensions like insulin and solids might be applied by this route.

Advantages

1. Absorption is slow and constant.

2. It is hygienic.

Disadvantages

1. It might lead to abscess formation.

2. Absorption is limited by blood flow.

Examples of drugs given by subcutaneous route include insulin, adrenaline and norplant.

b. Intramuscular Route: Intramuscular route might be applied to the buttock, thigh and deltoid. The volume used is 3 ml.

Advantages

1. Absorption is rapid than subcutaneous route.

2. Oily preparations can be used.

3. Irritative substances might be given.

4. Slow releasing drugs can be given by this route.

Disadvantages

Using this route might cause nerve or vein damage.

Intravenous Injections: Intravenous injections might be applied to the cubital, basilic and cephalic veins.

Advantages

1. Immediate action takes place.

2. This route is preferred in emergency situations.

3. This route is preferred for unconscious patients.

4. Titration of dose is possible.

5. Large volume of fluids might be injected by this route.

6. Diluted irritant might be injected.

7. Absorption is not required.

8. No first pass effect takes place.

9. Blood plasma or fluids might be injected.

Disadvantages

1. There is no retreat.

2. This method is more risky.

3. Sepsis-Infection might occur.

4. Phlebitis (Inflammation of the blood vessel) might occur.

5. Infiltration of surrounding tissues might result.

6. This method is not suitable for oily preparations.

7. This method is not suitable for insoluble preparations.

Intraarterial Route: This method is used for chemotherapy in cases of malignant tumors and in angiography.

Intradermal Route: This route is mostly used for diagnostic purposes and is involved in:

1. Schick test for Diphtheria.

2. Dick test for Scarlet fever.

3. Vaccines include DBT, BCG and polio.

4. Sensitivity is to penicillin.

Intracardiac Route: Injection can be applied to the left ventricle in case of cardiac arrest.

Intrathecal Route: Intrathecal route involves the subarachnoid space. Injection may be applied for the lumbar puncture, for spinal anesthesia and for diagnostic purposes.

This technique requires special precautions.

Intra-articular Route: Intra-articular route involves injection into the joint cavity. Corticosteroids may be injected by this route in acute arthritis.

Intraperitoneal Route: Intraperitoneal route may be used for peritoneal dialysis.

Intrapleural Route: Penicillin may be injected in cases of lung empyma by intrapleural route.

Injection into Bone Marrow: This route may be used for diagnostic or therapeutic purposes.

Hypospray/Jet Injection

This method is needleless and is subcutaneous done by applying pressure over the skin. The drug solution is retained under pressure in a container called 'gun'. It is held with nozzle against the skin. Pressure on the nozzle allows a fine jet of solution to emerge with great force. The solution can penetrate the skin and subcutaneous tissue to a variable depth as determined by the pressure. Mass inoculation is possible but the method is expensive, definite skills are required and cuts might result.

Inhalation

Inhalation may be the route of choice to avoid the systemic effects. In this way drugs can pass directly to the lungs. Drugs used involve volatile drugs and gases. Examples include aerosols like salbutamol; steam inhalations include tincture and Benzoin.

Advantages

1. Rapid absorption takes place.
2. Rapid onset of action takes place.
3. This route has minimum side effects.
4. No first pass effect takes place.
5. This method is easy.
6. Fewer doses is required.

Disadvantages

1. Special apparatus is required.
2. Irritation of the respiratory tract may take place.

3. Cooperation of the patient is required.

4. Airway must be patent.

Topical Route

Drugs may be applied to the external surfaces, the skin and the mucous membranes. Topical route includes:

a. Enepidermic Route: When the drug is applied to the outer skin, it is called enepidermic route of drug administration. Examples include poultices, plasters, creams and ointments.

b. Epidermic Route (Innunition): When the drug is rubbed into the skin, it is known as epidermic route. Examples include different oils.

c. Insufflations: When drug in finely powdered form is blown into the body cavities or spaces with special nebulizer, the method is known as insufflations.

d. Instillation: Liquids may be poured into the body by a dropper into the conjunctival sac, ear, nose and wounds. Solids may also be administered.

e. Irrigation or Douching: This method is used for washing a cavity e.g. urinary bladder, uterus, vagina and urethra. It is also used for application of antiseptic drugs.

f. Painting/Swabbing: Drugs are simply applied in the form of lotion on cutaneous or mucosal surfaces of buccal, nasal cavity and other internal organs.

Time of Action using Different Routes of Administration

Drugs take different time durations after injection using different routes to perform their actions. This time delay is important, oral route has controlled release time, thus depot or reservoir preparation may be made e.g. penicillin for rheumatic fever.

Usage of drug depends on its physical properties, chemical properties, speed of action, need and bypass effect.

References

- Maxmen A (2016). "Busting the billion-dollar myth: how to slash the cost of drug development". Nature. 536 (7617): 388–90. Bibcode:2016Natur.536..388M. Doi:10.1038/536388a. PMID 27558048

- Drug, terms: investopedia.com, Retrieved 21 July, 2019

- Anson D, Ma J, He JQ (1 May 2009). "Identifying Cardiotoxic Compounds". Genetic Engineering & Biotechnology News. Technote. 29 (9). Mary Ann Liebert. Pp. 34–35. ISSN 1935-472X. OCLC 77706455. Archived from the original on 21 September 2012. Retrieved 25 July 2009

- Sectionii, documents, nurses: dhhs.nh.gov, Retrieved 22 August, 2019

- Baños Díez, J. E.; March Pujol, M (2002). Farmacología ocular (in Spanish) (2da ed.). Edicions UPC. P. 87. ISBN 978-8483016473. Retrieved 23 May 2009

- Drug-classes-1123991: verywellhealth.com, Retrieved 23 January, 2019

- Herper, Matthew (11 August 2013). "The Cost Of Creating A New Drug Now $5 Billion, Pushing Big Pharma To Change". Forbes, Pharma & Healthcare. Retrieved 17 July2016

- Prescription-drugs, drug-facts: teens.drugabuse.gov, Retrieved 24 February, 2019

- Paul SM, Mytelka DS, Dunwiddie CT, Persinger CC, Munos BH, Lindborg SR, Schacht AL (March 2010). "How to improve R&D productivity: the pharmaceutical industry's grand challenge". Nature Reviews. Drug Discovery. 9 (3): 203–14. Doi:10.1038/nrd3078. PMID 20168317

- Routes-drug-administration, pharmacology: howmed.net, Retrieved 25 March, 2019

3

Pharmacokinetics

Pharmacokinetics is the branch of pharmacology which is concerned with determining the fate of the substances administered to a living organism. This chapter discusses in detail various aspects of pharmacokinetics including the absorption, distribution, metabolism and elimination of pharmaceutical drugs.

Pharmacokinetics is a fundamental scientific discipline that underpins applied therapeutics. Patients need to be prescribed appropriate medicines for a clinical condition. The medicine is chosen on the basis of an evidencebased approach to clinical practice and assured to be compatible with any other medicines or alternative therapies the patient may be taking.

The design of a dosage regimen is dependent on a basic understanding of the drug use process (DUP). When faced with a patient who shows specific clinical signs and symptoms, pharmacists must always ask a fundamental question: 'Is this patient suffering from a drug-related problem?' Once this issue is evaluated and a clinical diagnosis is available, the pharmacist can apply the DUP to ensure that the patient is prescribed an appropriate medication regimen, that the patient understands the therapy prescribed, and that an agreed concordance plan is achieved.

Pharmacists using the DUP consider:

- Need for a drug

- Choice of a drug

- Goals of therapy

- Design of regimen

  - Route

  - Dose and frequency

  - Duration

- Monitoring and review

- Counselling

Once a particular medicine is chosen, the principles of clinical pharmacokinetics are required to ensure the appropriate formulation of drug is chosen for an appropriate route of administration. On the basis of the patient's drug handling parameters, which require an understanding of absorption, distribution, metabolism and excretion, the dosage regimen for the medicine in a particular patient can be developed. The pharmacist will then need to ensure that the appropriate regimen is prescribed to achieve optimal efficacy and minimal toxicity. Pharmacists then ensure that the appropriate monitoring is undertaken and that the patient receives the appropriate information to ensure compliance. Clinical pharmacokinetics is thus a fundamental knowledge base that pharmacists require to ensure effective practice of pharmaceutical care.

Pharmacokinetics provides a mathematical basis to assess the time course of drugs and their effects in the body. It enables the following processes to be quantified:

- Absorption

- Distribution

- Metabolism

- Excretion

These pharmacokinetic processes, often referred to as ADME, determine the drug concentration in the body when medicines are prescribed. A fundamental understanding of these parameters is required to design an appropriate drug regimen for a patient. The effectiveness of a dosage regimen is determined by the concentration of the drug in the body.

Drugs that should be routinely monitored:

Therapeutic group	Drugs
Aminoglycosides	Gentamicin, tobramycin, amikacin
Cardioactive	Digoxin, lidocaine
Respiratory	Theophylline
Anticonvulsant	Phenytoin, carbamazepine, phenobarbital
Others	Lithium, ciclosporin

Ideally, the concentration of drug should be measured at the site of action of the drug; that is, at the receptor. However, owing to inaccessibility, drug concentrations are normally measured in whole blood from which serum or plasma is generated. Other body fluids such as saliva, urine and cerebrospinal fluid (CSF) are sometimes used. It is assumed that drug concentrations in these fluids are in equilibrium with the drug concentration at the receptor.

It should be noted that the measured drug concentrations in plasma or serum are often referred to as drug levels, which is the term that will be used throughout the text. It refers to total drug concentration, i.e. a combination of bound and free drug that are in equilibrium with each other.

In routine clinical practice, serum drug level monitoring and optimisation of a dosage regimen require the application of clinical pharmacokinetics. A number of drugs show a narrow therapeutic range and for these drugs therapeutic drug level monitoring is required. Table identifies drugs that should be routinely monitored.

A variety of techniques is available for representing the pharmacokinetics of a drug. The most usual is to view the body as consisting of compartments between which drug moves and from which elimination occurs. The transfer of drug between these compartments is represented by rate constants.

Rates of Reaction

To consider the processes of ADME the rates of these processes have to be considered; they can be characterised by two basic underlying concepts.

The rate of a reaction or process is defined as the velocity at which it proceeds and can be described as either zero-order or first-order.

Zero-order Reaction

Consider the rate of elimination of drug A from the body. If the amount of the drug, A, is decreasing at a constant rate, then the rate of elimination of A can be described as:

$$\frac{dA}{dt} = -k*$$

where $k*$ is the zero-order rate constant.

The reaction proceeds at a constant rate and is independent of the concentration of A present in the body. An example is the elimination of alcohol. Drugs that show this type of elimination will show accumulation of plasma levels of the drug and hence nonlinear pharmacokinetics.

First-Order Reaction

If the amount of drug A is decreasing at a rate that is proportional to A, the amount of drug A remaining in the body, then the rate of elimination of drug A can be described as:

$$\frac{dA}{dt} = -kA$$

where k is the first-order rate constant.

The reaction proceeds at a rate that is dependent on the concentration of A present in the body. It is assumed that the processes of ADME follow first-order reactions and most drugs are eliminated in this manner.

Most drugs used in clinical practice at therapeutic dosages will show first-order rate processes; that is, the rate of elimination of most drugs will be first-order. However, there are notable exceptions, for example phenytoin and high-dose salicylates. In essence, for drugs that show a first-order elimination process one can show that, as the amount of drug administered increases, the body is able to eliminate the drug accordingly and accumulation will not occur. If you double the dose you will double the plasma concentration. However, if you continue to increase the amount of drug administered then all drugs will change from showing a first-order process to a zero-order process, for example in an overdose situation.

ADME

ADME is an abbreviation in pharmacokinetics and pharmacology for "absorption, distribution, metabolism, and excretion", and describes the disposition of a pharmaceutical compound within an organism. The four criteria all influence the drug levels and kinetics of drug exposure to the tissues and hence influence the performance and pharmacological activity of the compound as a drug. Sometimes, liberation and/or toxicity are also considered, yielding LADME, ADMET, or LADMET.

Components

Absorption/Administration

For a compound to reach a tissue, it usually must be taken into the bloodstream - often via mucous surfaces like the digestive tract (intestinal absorption) - before being taken up by the target cells. Factors such as poor compound solubility, gastric emptying time, intestinal transit time, chemical instability in the stomach, and inability to permeate the intestinal wall can all reduce the extent to which a drug is absorbed after oral administration. Absorption critically determines the compound's bioavailability. Drugs that absorb poorly when taken orally must be administered in some less desirable way, like intravenously or by inhalation (e.g. zanamivir). Routes of administration are an important consideration.

Distribution

The compound needs to be carried to its effector site, most often via the bloodstream. From there, the compound may distribute into muscle and organs, usually to differing extents. After entry into the systemic circulation, either by intravascular injection or by absorption from any of the various extracellular sites, the drug is subjected to numerous distribution processes that tend to lower its plasma concentration.

Distribution is defined as the reversible transfer of a drug between one compartment to another. Some factors affecting drug distribution include regional blood flow rates, molecular size, polarity and binding to serum proteins, forming a complex. Distribution can be a serious problem at some natural barriers like the blood–brain barrier.

Metabolism

Compounds begin to break down as soon as they enter the body. The majority of small-molecule drug metabolism is carried out in the liver by redox enzymes, termed cytochrome P450 enzymes. As metabolism occurs, the initial (parent) compound is converted to new compounds called metabolites. When metabolites are pharmacologically inert, metabolism deactivates the administered dose of parent drug and this usually reduces the effects on the body. Metabolites may also be pharmacologically active, sometimes more so than the parent drug.

Excretion

Compounds and their metabolites need to be removed from the body via excretion, usually through the kidneys (urine) or in the feces. Unless excretion is complete, accumulation of foreign substances can adversely affect normal metabolism.

There are three main sites where drug excretion occurs. The kidney is the most important site and it is where products are excreted through urine. Biliary excretion or fecal excretion is the process that initiates in the liver and passes through to the gut until the products are finally excreted along with waste products or feces. The last main method of excretion is through the lungs (e.g. anesthetic gases).

Excretion of drugs by the kidney involves 3 main mechanisms:

- Glomerular filtration of unbound drug.
- Active secretion of (free & protein-bound) drug by transporters (e.g. anions such as urate, penicillin, glucuronide, sulfate conjugates) or cations such as choline, histamine.
- Filtrate 100-fold concentrated in tubules for a favorable concentration gradient so that it may be secreted by passive diffusion and passed out through the urine.

Toxicity

Sometimes, the potential or real toxicity of the compound is taken into account (ADME-Tox or ADMET). Parameters used to characterize toxicity include the median lethal dose (LD_{50}) and therapeutic index.

Computational chemists try to predict the ADME-Tox qualities of compounds through methods like QSPR or QSAR.

The route of administration critically influences ADME.

ABSORPTION OF PHARMACEUTICAL DRUGS

In pharmacology (and more specifically pharmacokinetics), absorption is the movement of a drug from the site of administration to bloodstream.

Absorption involves several phases. First, the drug needs to be introduced via some route of administration (oral, topical-dermal, etc.) and in a specific dosage form such as a tablet, capsule, solution and so on. Absorption depends upon the route of administration.

In other situations, such as intravenous therapy, intramuscular injection, enteral nutrition and others, absorption is even more straightforward and there is less variability in absorption and bioavailability is often near 100%. It is considered that intravascular administration (e.g. IV) does not involve absorption, and there is no loss of drug. The fastest route of absorption is inhalation, and not as mistakenly considered the intravenous administration.

Absorption is a primary focus in drug development and medicinal chemistry, since the drug must be absorbed before any medicinal effects can take place. Moreover, the drug's pharmacokinetic profile can be easily and significantly changed by adjusting factors that affect absorption.

Dissolution

In the most common situation, a tablet is ingested and passes through the esophagus to the stomach.

The rate of dissolution is a key target for controlling the duration of a drug's effect, and as such, several dosage forms that contain the same active ingredient may be available, differing only in the rate of dissolution. If a drug is supplied in a form that is not readily dissolved, the drug may be released more gradually over time with a longer duration of action. Having a longer duration of action may improve compliance since the medication will not have to be taken as often. Additionally, slow-release dosage forms may maintain concentrations within an acceptable therapeutic range over a long period of time, as opposed is quick-release dosage forms which may result in sharper peaks and troughs in serum concentrations.

The rate of dissolution is described by the Noyes–Whitney equation as shown below:

$$\frac{dW}{dt} = \frac{DA(C_s - C)}{L}$$

Where:

- $\dfrac{dW}{dt}$ is the rate of dissolution.

- A is the surface area of the solid.

- C is the concentration of the solid in the bulk dissolution medium.

- C_s is the concentration of the solid in the diffusion layer surrounding the solid.

- D is the diffusion coefficient.

- L is the diffusion layer thickness.

As can be inferred by the Noyes-Whitney equation, the rate of dissolution may be modified primarily by altering the surface area of the solid. The surface area may be adjusted by altering the particle size (e.g. micronization). For many drugs, reducing the particle size leads to a reduction in the dose that is required to achieve the same therapeutic effect. The reduction of particle size increases the specific surface area and the dissolution rate, and it does not affect solubility.

The rate of dissolution may also be altered by choosing a suitable polymorph of a compound. Different polymorphs exhibit different solubility and dissolution rate characteristics. Specifically, crystalline forms dissolve slower than amorphous forms, since crystalline forms require more energy to leave lattice during dissolution. The most stable crystalline polymorph has the lowest dissolution rate. Dissolution is also different for anhydrous and hydrous forms of a drug. Anhydrous often dissolve faster than hydrated; however, anhydrous forms sometimes exhibit lower solubility.

Chemical modification by esterification is also used to control solubility. For example, stearate and estolate esters of a drug have decreased solubility in gastric fluid. Later, esterases in the gastrointestinal tract (GIT) wall and blood hydrolyze these esters to release the parent drug.

Also, coatings on a tablet or a pellet may act as a barrier to reduce the rate of dissolution. Coating may also be used to modify where dissolution takes place. For example, enteric coatings may be applied to a drug, so that the coating only dissolves in the basic environment of the intestines. This will prevent release of the drug before reaching the intestines.

Since solutions are already dissolved, they do not need to undergo dissolution before being absorbed. Lipid-soluble drugs are less absorbed than water-soluble drugs, especially when they are enteral.

Ionization

The gastrointestinal tract is lined with epithelial cells. Drugs must pass or permeate through these cells in order to be absorbed into the circulatory system. One particular cellular barrier that may prevent absorption of a given drug is the cell membrane. Cell membranes are essentially lipid bilayers which form a semipermeable membrane. Pure lipid bilayers are generally permeable only to small, uncharged solutes. Hence, whether or not a molecule is ionized will affect its absorption, since ionic molecules are charged. Solubility favors charged species, and permeability favors neutral species. Some molecules have special exchange proteins and channels to facilitate movement from the lumen into the circulation.

Ions cannot passively diffuse through the gastrointestinal tract because the epithelial cell membrane is made up of a phospholipid bilayer. The bilayer is made up of two layers of phospholipids in which the charged hydrophilic heads face outwards and the non-charged hydrophobic fatty acid chains are in the middle of the layer. The uncharged fatty acid chains repel ionized, charged molecules. This means that the ionized molecules cannot pass through the intestinal membrane and be absorbed.

The Henderson-Hasselbalch equation offers a way to determine the proportion of a substance that is ionized at a given pH. In the stomach, drugs that are weak acids (such as aspirin) will be present mainly in their non-ionic form, and weak bases will be in their ionic form. Since non-ionic species diffuse more readily through cell membranes, weak acids will have a higher absorption in the highly acidic stomach.

However, the reverse is true in the basic environment of the intestines—weak bases (such as caffeine) will diffuse more readily since they will be non-ionic.

This aspect of absorption has been targeted by medicinal chemists. For example, a suitable analog may be chosen so that the drug is more likely to be in a non-ionic form. Also, prodrugs of a compound may be developed by medicinal chemists—these chemical variants may be more readily absorbed and then metabolized by the body into the active compound. However, changing the structure of a molecule is less predictable than altering dissolution properties, since changes in chemical structure may affect the pharmacodynamic properties of a drug.

Other Factors

Other facts that affect absorption include, but are not limited to, bioactivity, resonance, the inductive effect, isosterism, bio-isosterism, and consideration.

Bioavailability

In pharmacology, bioavailability (*BA or F*) is a subcategory of absorption and is the fraction of an administered dose of unchanged drug that reaches the systemic circulation, one of the principal pharmacokinetic properties of drugs. By definition, when a medication is administered intravenously, its bioavailability is 100%. However, when a medication is administered via other routes (such as orally), its bioavailability generally decreases (due to incomplete absorption and first-pass metabolism) or may vary from patient to patient.

Bioavailability is one of the essential tools in pharmacokinetics, as bioavailability must be considered when calculating dosages for non-intravenous routes of administration.

For dietary supplements, herbs and other nutrients in which the route of administration is nearly always oral, bioavailability generally designates simply the quantity or fraction of the ingested dose that is absorbed.

Bioavailability is defined slightly differently for drugs as opposed to dietary supplements primarily due to the method of administration and Food and Drug Administration regulations.

In Pharmacology

In pharmacology, bioavailability is a measurement of the rate and extent to which a drug reaches at the site of action. It is denoted by the letter f (or, if expressed in percent, by F).

In Nutritional Sciences

In nutritional sciences, which covers the intake of nutrients and non-drug dietary ingredients, the concept of bioavailability lacks the well-defined standards associated with the pharmaceutical industry. The pharmacological definition cannot apply to these substances because utilization and absorption is a function of the nutritional status and physiological state of the subject, resulting in even greater differences from individual to individual (inter-individual variation). Therefore, bioavailability for dietary supplements can be defined as the proportion of the administered substance capable of being absorbed and available for use or storage.

In both pharmacology and nutrition sciences, bioavailability is measured by calculating the area under curve (AUC) of the drug concentration time profile.

In Environmental Sciences or Science

Bioavailability is the measure by which various substances in the environment may enter into living organisms. It is commonly a limiting factor in the production of crops (due to solubility limitation or absorption of plant nutrients to soil colloids) and in the removal of toxic substances from the food chain by microorganisms (due to sorption to or partitioning of otherwise degradable substances into inaccessible phases in the environment). A noteworthy example for agriculture is plant phosphorus deficiency induced by precipitation with iron and aluminum phosphates at low soil pH and precipitation with calcium phosphates at high soil pH. Toxic materials in soil, such as lead from paint may be rendered unavailable to animals ingesting contaminated soil by supplying phosphorus fertilizers in excess. Organic pollutants such as solvents or pesticides may be rendered unavailable to microorganisms and thus persist in the environment when they are adsorbed to soil minerals or partition into hydrophobic organic matter.

Absolute Bioavailability

Absolute bioavailability compares the bioavailability of the active drug in systemic circulation following non-intravenous administration (i.e. after oral, ocular, rectal, transdermal, subcutaneous, or sublingual administration), with the bioavailability of the same drug following intravenous administration. It is the fraction of the drug absorbed through non-intravenous administration compared with the corresponding intravenous administration of the same drug. The comparison must be dose normalized (e.g. account for different doses or varying weights of the subjects); consequently, the amount absorbed is corrected by dividing the corresponding dose administered.

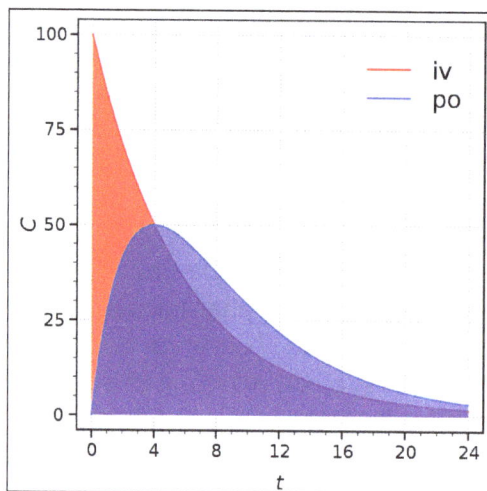

Absolute bioavailability is a ratio of areas under the curves. IV, intravenous; PO, oral route. C is plasma concentration (arbitrary units).

In pharmacology, in order to determine absolute bioavailability of a drug, a pharmacokinetic study must be done to obtain a plasma drug concentration vs time plot for the drug after both intravenous (iv) and extravascular (non-intravenous, i.e. oral) administration. The absolute bioavailability is the dose-corrected area under curve (AUC) non-intravenous divided by AUC intravenous. The formula for calculating the absolute bioavailability, F, of a drug administered orally (po) is given below (where D is dose administered).

$$F_{abs} = 100 \cdot \frac{AUC_{po} \cdot D_{iv}}{AUC_{iv} \cdot D_{po}}$$

Therefore, a drug given by the intravenous route will have an absolute bioavailability of 100% ($f = 1$), whereas drugs given by other routes usually have an absolute bioavailability of *less* than one. If we compare the two different dosage forms having same active ingredients and compare the two drug bioavailability is called comparative bioavailability.

Although knowing the true extent of systemic absorption (referred to as absolute bio-availability) is clearly useful, in practice it is not determined as frequently as one may think. The reason for this is that its assessment requires an intravenous reference; that is, a route of administration that guarantees all of the administered drug reaches systemic circulation. Such studies come at considerable cost, not least of which is the necessity to conduct preclinical toxicity tests to ensure adequate safety, as well as potential problems due to solubility limitations. These limitations may be overcome, however, by administering a very low dose (typically a few micrograms) of an isotopically labelled drug concomitantly with a therapeutic non-isotopically labelled oral dose (the isotopically-labelled intravenous dose is sufficiently low so as not to perturb the systemic drug concentrations achieved from the non-labelled oral dose). The intravenous and oral concentrations can then be deconvoluted by virtue of their different isotopic constitution, and can thus be used to determine the oral and intravenous pharmacokinetics from the same dose administration. This technique eliminates pharmacokinetic issues with non-equivalent clearance as well as enabling the intravenous dose to be administered with a minimum of toxicology and formulation. The technique was first applied using stable-isotopes such as ^{13}C and mass-spectrometry to distinguish the isotopes by mass difference. More recently, ^{14}C labelled drugs are administered intravenously and accelerator mass spectrometry (AMS) used to measure the isotopically labelled drug along with mass spectrometry for the unlabelled drug.

There is no regulatory requirement to define the intravenous pharmacokinetics or absolute bioavailability however regulatory authorities do sometimes ask for absolute bioavailability information of the extravascular route in cases in which the bioavailability is apparently low or variable and there is a proven relationship between the pharmacodynamics and the pharmacokinetics at therapeutic doses. In all such cases, to conduct an absolute bioavailability study requires that the drug be given intravenously.

Intravenous administration of a developmental drug can provide valuable information on the fundamental pharmacokinetic parameters of volume of distribution (V) and clearance (CL).

Relative Bioavailability and Bioequivalence

In pharmacology, relative bioavailability measures the bioavailability (estimated as the AUC) of a formulation (A) of a certain drug when compared with another formulation (B) of the same drug, usually an established standard, or through administration via a different route. When the standard consists of intravenously administered drug, this is known as absolute bioavailability.

$$F_{rel} = 100 \cdot \frac{AUC_A \cdot D_B}{AUC_B \cdot D_A}$$

Relative bioavailability is one of the measures used to assess bioequivalence (BE) between two drug products. For FDA approval, a generic manufacturer must demonstrate that the 90% confidence interval for the ratio of the mean responses (usually of AUC and the maximum concentration, C_{max}) of its product to that of the "brand name drug" is within the limits of 80% to 125%. Where AUC refers to the concentration of the drug in the blood over time $t = 0$ to $t = \infty$, C_{max} refers to the maximum concentration of the drug in the blood. When T_{max} is given, it refers to the time it takes for a drug to reach C_{max}.

While the mechanisms by which a formulation affects bioavailability and bioequivalence have been extensively studied in drugs, formulation factors that influence bioavailability and bioequivalence in nutritional supplements are largely unknown. As a result, in nutritional sciences, relative bioavailability or bioequivalence is the most common measure of bioavailability, comparing the bioavailability of one formulation of the same dietary ingredient to another.

Factors Influencing Bioavailability

The absolute bioavailability of a drug, when administered by an extravascular route, is usually less than one (i.e. $F < 100\%$). Various physiological factors reduce the availability of drugs prior to their entry into the systemic circulation. Whether a drug is taken with or without food will also affect absorption, other drugs taken concurrently may alter absorption and first-pass metabolism, intestinal motility alters the dissolution of the drug and may affect the degree of chemical degradation of the drug by intestinal microflora. Disease states affecting liver metabolism or gastrointestinal function will also have an effect.

Other factors may include, but are not limited to:

- Physical properties of the drug (hydrophobicity, pKa, solubility).
- The drug formulation (immediate release, excipients used, manufacturing methods, modified release – delayed release, extended release, sustained release, etc).
- Whether the formulation is administered in a fed or fasted state.
- Gastric emptying rate.
- Circadian differences.
- Interactions with other drugs/foods:
  - Interactions with other drugs (e.g. antacids, alcohol, nicotine).
  - Interactions with other foods (e.g. grapefruit juice, pomello, cranberry juice, brassica vegetables.
- Transporters: Substrate of efflux transporters (e.g. P-glycoprotein).
- Health of the gastrointestinal tract.

- Enzyme induction/inhibition by other drugs/foods:

  ∘ Enzyme induction (increased rate of metabolism), e.g. Phenytoin induces CYP1A2, CYP2C9, CYP2C19, and CYP3A4.

  ∘ Enzyme inhibition (decreased rate of metabolism), e.g. grapefruit juice inhibits CYP3A → higher nifedipine concentrations.

- Individual variation in metabolic differences:

  ∘ Age: In general, drugs are metabolized more slowly in fetal, neonatal, and geriatric populations.

  ∘ Phenotypic differences, enterohepatic circulation, diet, gender.

- Disease state:

  ∘ E.g. hepatic insufficiency, poor renal function.

Each of these factors may vary from patient to patient (inter-individual variation), and indeed in the same patient over time (intra-individual variation). In clinical trials, inter-individual variation is a critical measurement used to assess the bioavailability differences from patient to patient in order to ensure predictable dosing.

Bioavailability of Drugs versus Dietary Supplements

In comparison to drugs, there are significant differences in dietary supplements that impact the evaluation of their bioavailability. These differences include the following: the fact that nutritional supplements provide benefits that are variable and often qualitative in nature; the measurement of nutrient absorption lacks the precision; nutritional supplements are consumed for prevention and well-being; nutritional supplements do not exhibit characteristic dose-response curves; and dosing intervals of nutritional supplements, therefore, are not critical in contrast to drug therapy.

In addition, the lack of defined methodology and regulations surrounding the consumption of dietary supplements hinders the application of bioavailability measures in comparison to drugs. In clinical trials with dietary supplements, bioavailability primarily focuses on statistical descriptions of mean or average AUC differences between treatment groups, while often failing to compare or discuss their standard deviations or inter-individual variation. This failure leaves open the question of whether or not an individual in a group is likely to experience the benefits described by the mean-difference comparisons. it would be difficult to communicate meaning of these inter-subject variances to consumers and/or their physicians.

Nutritional Science: Reliable and Universal Bioavailability

One way to resolve this problem is to define "reliable bioavailability" as positive bioavailability results (an absorption meeting a predefined criterion) that include 84%

of the trial subjects and universal bioavailability as those that include 98% of the trial subjects. This reliable-universal framework would improve communications with physicians and consumers such that, if it were included on products labels for example, make educated choices as to the benefits of a formulation for them directly. In addition, the reliable-universal framework is similar to the construction of confidence intervals, which statisticians have long offered as one potential solution for dealing with small samples, violations of statistical assumptions or large standard deviations.

DISTRIBUTION OF PHARMACEUTICAL DRUGS

Distribution in pharmacology is a branch of pharmacokinetics which describes the reversible transfer of a drug from one location to another within the body.

Once a drug enters into systemic circulation by absorption or direct administration, it must be distributed into interstitial and intracellular fluids. Each organ or tissue can receive different doses of the drug and the drug can remain in the different organs or tissues for a varying amount of time. The distribution of a drug between tissues is dependent on vascular permeability, regional blood flow, cardiac output and perfusion rate of the tissue and the ability of the drug to bind tissue and plasma proteins and its lipid solubility. pH partition plays a major role as well. The drug is easily distributed in highly perfused organs such as the liver, heart and kidney. It is distributed in small quantities through less perfused tissues like muscle, fat and peripheral organs. The drug can be moved from the plasma to the tissue until the equilibrium is established (for unbound drug present in plasma).

The concept of compartmentalization of an organism must be considered when discussing a drug's distribution. This concept is used in pharmacokinetic modelling.

Factors that affect Distribution

There are many factors that affect a drug's distribution throughout an organism, but Pascuzzo considers that the most important ones are the following: an organism's physical volume, the removal rate and the degree to which a drug binds with plasma proteins and/or tissues.

Physical Volume of an Organism

This concept is related to multi-compartmentalization. Any drugs within an organism will act as a solute and the organism's tissues will act as solvents. The differing specificities of different tissues will give rise to different concentrations of the drug within each group. Therefore, the chemical characteristics of a drug will determine its distribution within an organism. For example, a liposoluble drug will tend to accumulate in body fat and water-soluble drugs will tend to accumulate in extracellular fluids. The volume of distribution (V_D) of a drug is a property that quantifies the extent of its distribution. It can be defined as the theoretical volume that a drug would have to occupy (if it were uniformly distributed), to provide the same concentration as it currently is in blood plasma. It can be determined from the following formula: $Vd = \dfrac{Ab}{Cp}$ Where: Ab is total amount of the drug in the body and is the drug's plasma concentration.

As the value for Ab is equivalent to the dose of the drug that has been administered the formula shows us that there is an inversely proportional relationship between Vd and Cp .That is, that the greater Cp is the lower Vd will be and vice versa. It therefore follows that the factors that increase Cp will decrease Vd . This gives an indication of the importance of knowledge relating to the drug's plasma concentration and the factors that modify it.

If this formula is applied to the concepts relating to bioavailability, we can calculate the amount of drug to administer in order to obtain a required concentration of the drug in the organism (*loading dose*):

$$Dc = \frac{Vd.Cp}{Da.B}$$

This concept is of clinical interest as it is sometimes necessary to reach a certain concentration of a drug that is known to be optimal in order for it to have the required effects on the organism (as occurs if a patient is to be scanned).

Removal Rate

A drug's removal rate will be determined by the proportion of the drug that is removed from circulation by each organ once the drug has been delivered to the organ by the circulating blood supply. This new concept builds on earlier ideas and it depends on a number of distinct factors:

- The drugs characteristics, including its pKa.

- Redistribution through an organism's tissues: Some drugs are distributed rapidly in some tissues until they reach equilibrium with the plasma concentration. However, other tissues with a slower rate of distribution will continue to absorb the drug from the plasma over a longer period. This will mean that the drug concentration in the first tissue will be greater than the plasma concentration and the drug will move from the tissue back into the plasma. This phenomenon will continue until the drug has reached equilibrium over the whole organism. The most sensitive tissue will therefore experience two different drug concentrations: an initial higher concentration and a later lower concentration as a consequence of tissue redistribution.

- Concentration differential between tissues.

- Exchange surface.

- Presence of natural barriers. These are obstacles to a drug's diffusion similar to those encountered during its absorption. The most interesting are:

  ○ Capillary bed permeability, which varies between tissues.

  ○ Blood-brain barrier: This is located between the blood plasma in the cerebral blood vessels and the brain's extracellular space. The presence of this barrier makes it hard for a drug to reach the brain.

  ○ Placental barrier: This prevents high concentrations of a potentially toxic drug from reaching the foetus.

Plasma Protein Binding

Some drugs have the capacity to bind with certain types of proteins that are carried in blood plasma. This is important as only drugs that are present in the plasma in their free form can be transported to the tissues. Drugs that are bound to plasma proteins therefore act as a reservoir of the drug within the organism and this binding reduces the drug's final concentration in the tissues. The binding between a drug and plasma protein is rarely specific and is usually labile and reversible. The binding generally involves ionic bonds, hydrogen bonds, Van der Waals forces and, less often, covalent bonds. This means that the bond between a drug and a protein can be broken and the drug can be replaced by another substance (or another drug) and that, regardless of this, the protein binding is subject to saturation. An equilibrium also exists between the free drug in the blood plasma and that bound to proteins, meaning that the proportion of the drug bound to plasma proteins will be stable, independent of its total concentration in the plasma.

In vitro studies carried out under optimum conditions have shown that the equilibrium between a drug's plasmatic concentration and its tissue concentration is only significantly altered at binding rates to plasma proteins of greater than 90%. Above these levels the drug is sequestered, which decreases its presence in tissues by up to 50%. This is important when considering pharmacological interactions: the tissue concentration of a drug with a plasma protein binding rate of less than 90% is not going to significantly increase if that drug is displaced from its union with a protein by another substance. On the other hand, at binding rates of greater than 95% small changes can cause important modifications in a drug's tissue concentration. This will, in turn, increase the risk of the drug having a toxic effect on tissues.

Perhaps the most important plasma proteins are the albumins as they are present in relatively high concentrations and they readily bind to other substances. Other important proteins include the glycoproteins, the lipoproteins and to a lesser degree the globulins.

It is therefore easy to see that clinical conditions that modify the levels of plasma proteins (for example, hypoalbuminemias brought on by renal dysfunction) may affect the effect and toxicity of a drug that has a binding rate with plasma proteins of above 90%.

Redistribution

Highly lipid-soluble drugs given by intravenous or inhalation routes are initially distributed to organs with high blood flow. Later, less vascular but more bulky tissues (such as muscle and fat) take up the drug—plasma concentration falls and the drug is withdrawn from these sites. If the site of action of the drug was in one of the highly perfused organs, redistribution results in termination of the drug action. The greater the lipid solubility of the drug, the faster its redistribution will be. For example, the anaesthetic action of thiopentone is terminated in a few minutes due to redistribution. However, when the same drug is given repeatedly or continuously over long periods, the low-perfusion and high-capacity sites are progressively filled up and the drug becomes longer-acting.

It is reversible process of moving drug of sites of highly perfused to systemic circulation, FMAS.

METABOLISM OF PHARMACEUTICAL DRUGS

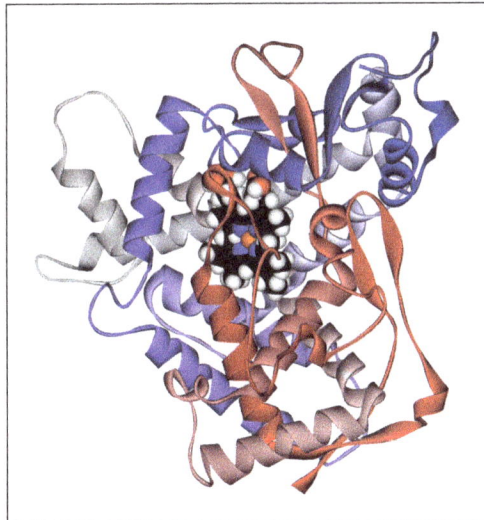

Cytochrome P450 oxidases are important enzymes in xenobiotic metabolism.

Drug metabolism is the metabolic breakdown of drugs by living organisms, usually through specialized enzymatic systems. More generally, xenobiotic metabolism is the set of metabolic pathways that modify the chemical structure of xenobiotics, which are compounds foreign to an organism's normal biochemistry, such as any drug or poison. These pathways are a form of biotransformation present in all major groups of organisms, and are considered to be of ancient origin. These reactions often act to detoxify poisonous compounds (although in some cases the intermediates in xenobiotic metabolism can themselves cause toxic effects). The study of drug metabolism is called pharmacokinetics.

The metabolism of pharmaceutical drugs is an important aspect of pharmacology and medicine. For example, the rate of metabolism determines the duration and intensity of a drug's pharmacologic action. Drug metabolism also affects multidrug resistance in infectious diseases and in chemotherapy for cancer, and the actions of some drugs as substrates or inhibitors of enzymes involved in xenobiotic metabolism are a common reason for hazardous drug interactions. These pathways are also important in environmental science, with the xenobiotic metabolism of microorganisms determining whether a pollutant will be broken down during bioremediation, or persist in the environment. The enzymes of xenobiotic metabolism, particularly the glutathione S-transferases are also important in agriculture, since they may produce resistance to pesticides and herbicides.

Drug metabolism is divided into three phases. In phase I, enzymes such as cytochrome P450 oxidases introduce reactive or polar groups into xenobiotics. These modified compounds are then conjugated to polar compounds in phase II reactions. These reactions are catalysed by transferase enzymes such as glutathione S-transferases. Finally, in phase III, the conjugated xenobiotics may be further processed, before being recognised by efflux transporters and pumped out of cells. Drug metabolism often converts lipophilic compounds into hydrophilic products that are more readily excreted.

Permeability Barriers and Detoxification

The exact compounds an organism is exposed to will be largely unpredictable, and may differ widely over time; these are major characteristics of xenobiotic toxic stress. The major challenge faced by xenobiotic detoxification systems is that they must be able to remove the almost-limitless number of xenobiotic compounds from the complex mixture of chemicals involved in normal metabolism. The solution that has evolved to address this problem is an elegant combination of physical barriers and low-specificity enzymatic systems.

All organisms use cell membranes as hydrophobic permeability barriers to control access to their internal environment. Polar compounds cannot diffuse across these cell membranes, and the uptake of useful molecules is mediated through transport proteins that specifically select substrates from the extracellular mixture. This selective uptake means that most hydrophilic molecules cannot enter cells, since they are not recognised by any specific transporters. In contrast, the diffusion of hydrophobic compounds across these barriers cannot be controlled, and organisms, therefore, cannot exclude lipid-soluble xenobiotics using membrane barriers.

However, the existence of a permeability barrier means that organisms were able to evolve detoxification systems that exploit the hydrophobicity common to membrane-permeable xenobiotics. These systems therefore solve the specificity problem by possessing such broad substrate specificities that they metabolise almost any non-polar compound. Useful metabolites are excluded since they are polar, and in general contain one or more charged groups.

The detoxification of the reactive by-products of normal metabolism cannot be achieved by the systems outlined above, because these species are derived from normal cellular constituents and usually share their polar characteristics. However, since these compounds are few in number, specific enzymes can recognize and remove them. Examples of these specific detoxification systems are the glyoxalase system, which removes the reactive aldehyde methylglyoxal, and the various antioxidant systems that eliminate reactive oxygen species.

Phases of Detoxification

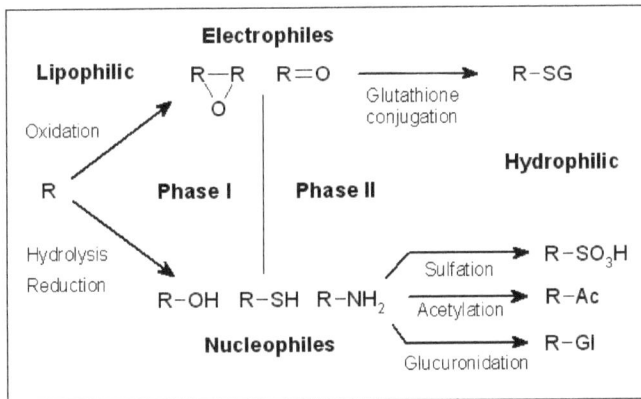

Phases I and II of the metabolism of a lipophilic xenobiotic.

The metabolism of xenobiotics is often divided into three phases:- modification, conjugation, and excretion. These reactions act in concert to detoxify xenobiotics and remove them from cells.

Phase I – Modification

In phase I, a variety of enzymes act to introduce reactive and polar groups into their substrates. One of the most common modifications is hydroxylation catalysed by the cytochrome P-450-dependent mixed-function oxidase system. These enzyme complexes act to incorporate an atom of oxygen into nonactivated hydrocarbons, which can result in either the introduction of hydroxyl groups or N-, O- and S-dealkylation of substrates. The reaction mechanism of the P-450 oxidases proceeds through the reduction of cytochrome-bound oxygen and the generation of a highly-reactive oxyferryl species, according to the following scheme:

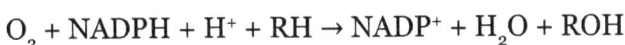

$$O_2 + NADPH + H^+ + RH \rightarrow NADP^+ + H_2O + ROH$$

Phase I reactions (also termed nonsynthetic reactions) may occur by oxidation, reduction, hydrolysis, cyclization, decyclization, and addition of oxygen or removal of hydrogen, carried out by mixed function oxidases, often in the liver. These oxidative reactions typically involve a cytochrome P450 monooxygenase (often abbreviated CYP), NADPH and oxygen. The classes of pharmaceutical drugs that utilize this method for their metabolism include phenothiazines, paracetamol, and steroids. If the metabolites of phase I reactions are sufficiently polar, they may be readily excreted at this point. However, many phase I products are not eliminated rapidly and undergo a subsequent reaction in which an endogenous substrate combines with the newly incorporated functional group to form a highly polar conjugate.

A common Phase I oxidation involves conversion of a C-H bond to a C-OH. This reaction sometimes converts a pharmacologically inactive compound (a prodrug) to a pharmacologically active one. By the same token, Phase I can turn a nontoxic molecule into a poisonous one (toxification). Simple hydrolysis in the stomach is normally an innocuous reaction, however there are exceptions. For example, phase I metabolism converts acetonitrile to $HOCH_2CN$, which rapidly dissociates into formaldehyde and hydrogen cyanide.

Phase I metabolism of drug candidates can be simulated in the laboratory using non-enzyme catalysts. This example of a biomimetic reaction tends to give products that often contains the Phase I metabolites. As an example, the major metabolite of the pharmaceutical trimebutine, desmethyltrimebutine (nor-trimebutine), can be efficiently produced by in vitro oxidation of the commercially available drug. Hydroxylation of an N-methyl group leads to expulsion of a molecule of formaldehyde, while oxidation of the O-methyl groups takes place to a lesser extent.

Oxidation

- Cytochrome P450 monooxygenase system.

- Flavin-containing monooxygenase system.

- Alcohol dehydrogenase and aldehyde dehydrogenase.

- Monoamine oxidase.

- Co-oxidation by peroxidases.

Reduction

- NADPH-cytochrome P450 reductase: Cytochrome P450 reductase, also known as NADPH:ferrihemoprotein oxidoreductase, NADPH:hemoprotein oxidoreductase, NADPH:P450 oxidoreductase, P450 reductase, POR, CPR, CYPOR, is a membrane-bound enzyme required for electron transfer to cytochrome P450 in the microsome of the eukaryotic cell from a FAD- and

FMN-containing enzyme NADPH:cytochrome P450 reductase. The general scheme of electron flow in the POR/P450 system is: NADPH → FAD → FMN → P450 → O_2.

- Reduced (ferrous) cytochrome P450: During reduction reactions, a chemical can enter futile cycling, in which it gains a free-radical electron, then promptly loses it to oxygen (to form a superoxide anion).

Hydrolysis

- Esterases and amidase.

- Epoxide hydrolase.

Phase II – Conjugation

In subsequent phase II reactions, these activated xenobiotic metabolites are conjugated with charged species such as glutathione (GSH), sulfate, glycine, or glucuronic acid. Sites on drugs where conjugation reactions occur include carboxyl (-COOH), hydroxyl (-OH), amino (NH_2), and sulfhydryl (-SH) groups. Products of conjugation reactions have increased molecular weight and tend to be less active than their substrates, unlike Phase I reactions which often produce active metabolites. The addition of large anionic groups (such as GSH) detoxifies reactive electrophiles and produces more polar metabolites that cannot diffuse across membranes, and may, therefore, be actively transported.

These reactions are catalysed by a large group of broad-specificity transferases, which in combination can metabolise almost any hydrophobic compound that contains nucleophilic or electrophilic groups. One of the most important classes of this group is that of the glutathione S-transferases (GSTs).

Mechanism	Involved enzyme	Co-factor	Location
Methylation	Methyltransferase	S-adenosyl-L-methionine	Liver, kidney, lung, CNS
Sulphation	Sulfotransferases	3'-phosphoadenosine-5'-phosphosulfate	Liver, kidney, intestine
Acetylation	• N-acetyltransferases • Bile acid-CoA:amino acid N-acyltransferases	acetyl coenzyme A	Liver, lung, spleen, gastric mucosa, RBCs, lymphocytes
Glucuronidation	UDP-glucuronosyltransferases	UDP-glucuronic acid	Liver, kidney, intestine, lung, skin, prostate, brain
Glutathione conjugation	Glutathione S-transferases	Glutathione	Liver, kidney

glycine conjuga- tion	Two step process: 1. XM-ligase (forms a xenobiotic acyl-CoA) 2. Glycine N-acyltrans- ferase (forms the glycine conjugate)	glycine	liver, kidney

Phase III – Further Modification and Excretion

After phase II reactions, the xenobiotic conjugates may be further metabolised. A common example is the processing of glutathione conjugates to acetylcysteine (mercapturic acid) conjugates. Here, the γ-glutamate and glycine residues in the glutathione molecule are removed by Gamma-glutamyl transpeptidase and dipeptidases. In the final step, the cystine residue in the conjugate is acetylated.

Conjugates and their metabolites can be excreted from cells in phase III of their metabolism, with the anionic groups acting as affinity tags for a variety of membrane transporters of the multidrug resistance protein (MRP) family. These proteins are members of the family of ATP-binding cassette transporters and can catalyse the ATP-dependent transport of a huge variety of hydrophobic anions, and thus act to remove phase II products to the extracellular medium, where they may be further metabolised or excreted.

Endogenous Toxins

The detoxification of endogenous reactive metabolites such as peroxides and reactive aldehydes often cannot be achieved by the system. This is the result of these species' being derived from normal cellular constituents and usually sharing their polar characteristics. However, since these compounds are few in number, it is possible for enzymatic systems to utilize specific molecular recognition to recognize and remove them. The similarity of these molecules to useful metabolites therefore means that different detoxification enzymes are usually required for the metabolism of each group of endogenous toxins. Examples of these specific detoxification systems are the glyoxalase system, which acts to dispose of the reactive aldehyde methylglyoxal, and the various antioxidant systems that remove reactive oxygen species.

Sites

Quantitatively, the smooth endoplasmic reticulum of the liver cell is the principal organ of drug metabolism, although every biological tissue has some ability to metabolize drugs. Factors responsible for the liver's contribution to drug metabolism include that it is a large organ, that it is the first organ perfused by chemicals absorbed in the gut, and that there are very high concentrations of most drug metabolizing enzyme systems relative to other organs. If a drug is taken into the GI tract, where it enters hepatic circulation through the portal vein, it becomes well-metabolized and is said to show the first pass effect.

Other sites of drug metabolism include epithelial cells of the gastrointestinal tract, lungs, kidneys, and the skin. These sites are usually responsible for localized toxicity reactions.

Factors that affect Drug Metabolism

The duration and intensity of pharmacological action of most lipophilic drugs are determined by the rate they are metabolized to inactive products. The Cytochrome P450 monooxygenase system is the most important pathway in this regard. In general, anything that increases the rate of metabolism (e.g. enzyme induction) of a pharmacologically active metabolite will decrease the duration and intensity of the drug action. The opposite is also true (e.g. enzyme inhibition). However, in cases where an enzyme is responsible for metabolizing a pro-drug into a drug, enzyme induction can speed up this conversion and increase drug levels, potentially causing toxicity.

Various physiological and pathological factors can also affect drug metabolism. Physiological factors that can influence drug metabolism include age, individual variation (e.g. pharmacogenetics), enterohepatic circulation, nutrition, intestinal flora, or sex differences.

In general, drugs are metabolized more slowly in fetal, neonatal and elderly humans and animals than in adults.

Genetic variation (polymorphism) accounts for some of the variability in the effect of drugs. With N-acetyltransferases (involved in Phase II reactions), individual variation creates a group of people who acetylate slowly (slow acetylators) and those who acetylate quickly, split roughly 50:50 in the population of Canada. This variation may have dramatic consequences, as the slow acetylators are more prone to dose-dependent toxicity.

Cytochrome P450 monooxygenase system enzymes can also vary across individuals, with deficiencies occurring in 1 – 30% of people, depending on their ethnic background.

Dose, frequency, route of administration, tissue distribution and protein binding of the drug affect its metabolism.

Pathological factors can also influence drug metabolism, including liver, kidney, or heart diseases.

In silico modelling and simulation methods allow drug metabolism to be predicted in virtual patient populations prior to performing clinical studies in human subjects. This can be used to identify individuals most at risk from adverse reaction.

ELIMINATION OF PHARMACEUTICAL DRUGS

In pharmacology the elimination or excretion of a drug is understood to be any one of a number of processes by which a drug is eliminated (that is, cleared and excreted) from an organism either in an unaltered form (unbound molecules) or modified as a metabolite. The kidney is the main excretory organ although others exist such as the liver, the skin, the lungs or glandular structures, such as the salivary glands and the lacrimal glands. These organs or structures use specific routes to expel a drug from the body, these are termed elimination pathways:

- Urine
- Tears
- Perspiration
- Saliva

- Respiration
- Milk
- Faeces
- Bile

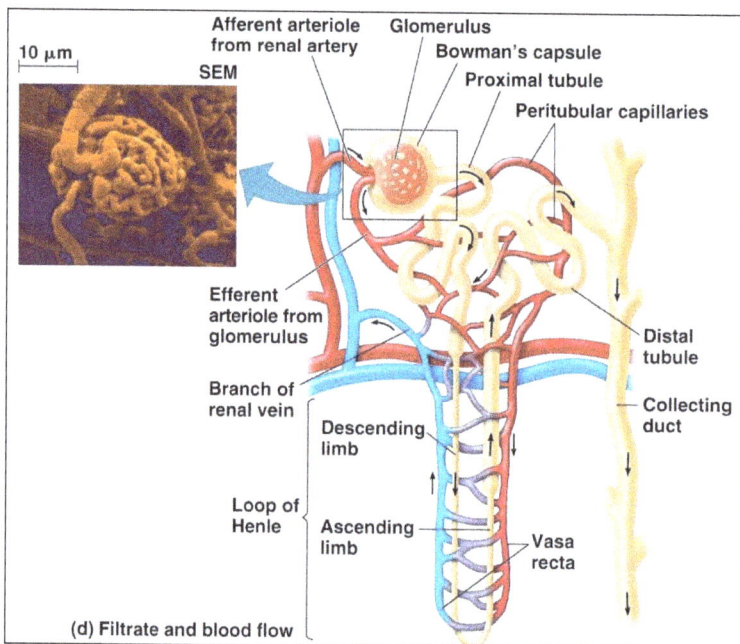

Diagram illustrating renal flow along the nephron.

Drugs are excreted from the kidney by glomerular filtration and by active tubular secretion following the same steps and mechanisms as the products of intermediate metabolism. Therefore, drugs that are filtered by the glomerulus are also subject to the process of passive tubular reabsorption. Glomerular filtration will only remove those drugs or metabolites that are not bound to proteins present in blood plasma (free fraction) and many other types of drugs (such as the organic acids) are actively secreted. In the proximal and distal convoluted tubules non-ionised acids and weak bases are reabsorbed both actively and passively. Weak acids are excreted when the tubular fluid becomes too alkaline and this reduces passive reabsorption. The opposite occurs with weak bases. Poisoning treatments use this effect to increase elimination, by alkalizing the urine causing forced diuresis which promotes excretion of a weak acid, rather than it getting reabsorbed. As the acid is ionised, it cannot pass through the plasma membrane back into the blood stream and instead gets excreted with the urine. Acidifying the urine has the same effect for weakly basic drugs.

On other occasions drugs combine with bile juices and enter the intestines. In the intestines the drug will join with the unabsorbed fraction of the administered dose and be eliminated with the faeces or it may undergo a new process of absorption to eventually be eliminated by the kidney.

The other elimination pathways are less important in the elimination of drugs, except in very specific cases, such as the respiratory tract for alcohol or anaesthetic gases. The case of mother's milk is of special importance. The liver and kidneys of newly born infants are relatively undeveloped and they are highly sensitive to a drug's toxic effects. For this reason it is important to know if a drug is likely to be eliminated from a woman's body if she is breast feeding in order to avoid this situation.

Pharmacokinetic Parameters of Elimination

Pharmacokinetics studies the manner and speed with which drugs and their metabolites are eliminated by the various excretory organs. This elimination will be proportional to the drug's plasmatic concentrations. In order to model these processes a working definition is required for some of the concepts related to excretion.

Half Life

The plasma half-life or *half life of elimination* is the time required to eliminate 50% of the absorbed dose of a drug from an organism. Or put another way, the time that it takes for the plasma concentration to fall by half from its maximum levels.

Clearance

The difference in a drug's concentration in arterial blood (before it has circulated around the body) and venous blood (after it has passed through the body's organs) represents the amount of the drug that the body has eliminated or cleared. Although clearance may also involve other organs than the kidney, it is almost synonymous with renal clearance or renal plasma clearance. Clearance is therefore expressed as the plasma volume totally free of the drug per unit of time, and it is measured in units of volume per units of time. Clearance can be determined on an overall, organism level ("systemic clearance") or at an organ level (hepatic clearance, renal clearance etc.). The equation that describes this concept is:

$$CL_o = Q \cdot \frac{(C_A - C_V)}{C_A}$$

Where CL_o is the organ's clearance rate, C_A is the drug's plasma concentration in arterial blood, C_V is the drug's plasma concentration in venous blood and Q an organ's blood flow.

Each organ will have its own specific clearance conditions, which will relate to its mode of action. The renal clearance rate will be determined by factors such as the degree of plasma protein binding as the drug will only be filtered out if it is in the unbound free form, the degree of saturation of the transporters (active secretion depends on transporter proteins that can become saturated) or the number of functioning nephrons (hence the importance of factors such as renal failure).

As hepatic clearance is an active process it is therefore determined by factors that alter an organism's metabolism such as the number of functioning hepatocytes, this is the reason that liver failure has such clinical importance.

Steady State

The steady state or stable concentration is reached when the drug's supply to the blood plasma is the same as the rate of elimination from the plasma. It is necessary to calculate this concentration in order to decide the period between doses and the amount of drug supplied with each dose in prolonged treatments.

Other Parameters

Other parameters of interest include a drug's bioavailability and the apparent volume of distribution.

PHARMACOKINETIC MODELS

Drugs remain in dynamic state within the body and drug events often happen simultaneously. In order to describe a complex biologic system, assumptions are made concerning the movement of drugs. The mathematical models are used to describe the absorption, distribution and elimination of drugs.

Mathematical equations are used to describe the drug concentration in the body as a function of time. For example, if the drug is administered (i.v.) it is distributed rapidly in the body fluid. The pharmacokinetic model that will describe this situation would be a tank containing a volume of fluid which is rapidly equilibrated with the drug. In the animals body a fraction of drug is continuously eliminated as function of time.

The concentration of a drug after a given dose in governed by two important parameters:

1. The fluid volume of the body.

2. The elimination of drug in unit time.

In pharmacokinetics the above parameters are assumed to be constants. If a known set of drug concentrations in the body is determined at various time intervals then the volume of the body fluid and the rate of drug elimination is established.

Types of Pharmacokinetic Models

Compartment Models

Similar to humans, the animal body is considered as a series of compartments. Each compartment communicate each other reversibly. A compartment is not a real anatomic region but a group of tissues which have similar blood flow. Within each compartment drug is distributed uniformly. Drugs move in and out of the compartment.

Rate constants K_{12} and K_{21} are used to represent the constants for transfer of drug from central to peripheral and from peripheral to central compartment respectively. The model is called open model because the drug can be eliminated.

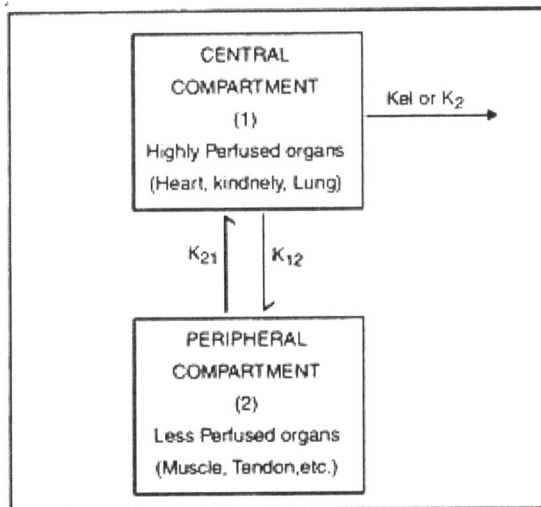

Schematic representation of compartment model showing
central (1) and peripheral (2) compartments.

Central Compartment

The well perfused tissues like liver, kidney and heart make the central compartment.

Peripheral Compartment

The peripheral compartment consists of the less perfused tissues like skin, bone, cartilages etc. The brain and bones as well as other parts of the central nervous system is excluded, since most drugs have little penetration into these organs. The sketch diagram of the pharmacokinetic model.

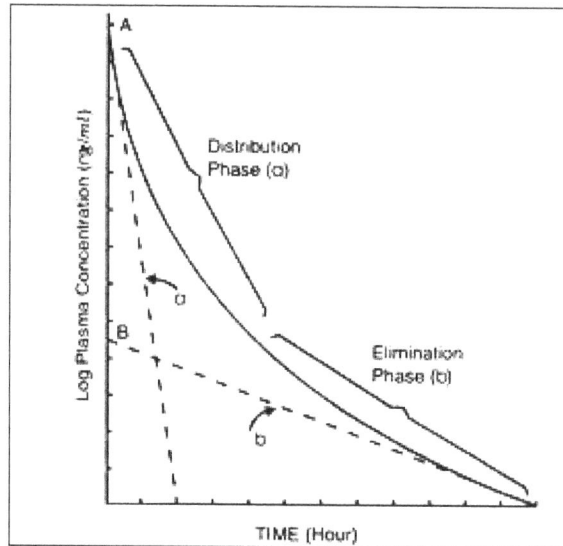

Semilogarithmic, plasma level time-curve for two-compartment model showing Distribution (a) and Elimination Phase (6) after single Iv. dose administration.

One Compartment Open Model

When a drug is given as rapid i.v. bolus, the entire dose of the drug enters the body immediately. In this case, the rate of absorption is neglected in calculations. In most cases the drug distributes via the circulation to all the tissues in the body.

The most simple pharmacokinetic model for describing the dissolution of the drug is an apparent volume within the body. The one compartment model assumes that any change in the plasma levels of drug reflects proportional changes in tissues drug concentrations.

Two Compartment Open Model

In this model it is assumed that the drug is distributed in two compartments. If drug is administered in animals body through i.v. injection, it is first distributed into the highly perfused tissues (central compartment) and thereafter to less perfused tissues (peripheral compartment). If plasma level-time profile is plotted on semi-logarithmic graph it gives a bi-exponential appearance.

Why a Steep Decline is Obtained?

After an i.v injection of a drug, concentrations in plasma decline rapidly because of drug distribution into peripheral compartment and the bi-exponential curve shows a steep line initially.

Distribution (α) and elimination (β) Phases: The initial steep decline of a drug concentration in central compartment is known as distribution phase (α) of the curve. In time, the drug attains a state of equilibrium between the central compartment and the peripheral compartment.

After this equilibrium is established, the loss of the drug from the central compartment appears to be a single first-order process due to overall process of elimination of the drug from the body. This second, lower rate process is known as the elimination phase (β).

The theoretical tissue compartment of a drug can be calculated once the parameters for the model are determined. The drug concentration in the tissue compartment represents the average drug concentration in a group of tissues rather than any real anatomic tissue drug concentration.

Real tissue drug concentration can sometimes be calculated by the addition of compartments to the model unit. In-spite of the hypothetical nature of the tissue compartment the theoretical tissue level is still a valuable piece of information for clinicians.

Why Initial Experimental Samples are Essential

In practice, samples of blood are removed from the central compartment and analyzed for the presence of drug. The plasma concentration time-curve represents distribution phase (α) followed by an elimination phase (β) after the tissue compartment has also been diffused with the drug.

The distribution phase may take minutes and may be missed entirely if the blood is sampled too late after administration of the drug. This is why the blood samples are collected initially starting from 2 min. or even earlier than this.

The following equations describe the change in drug concentration in plasma and in the tissue with respect to time:

$$Cp = \frac{D}{V_p}\left[\frac{K_{21}-\alpha}{\beta-\alpha}\right]e^{-\alpha t} + \left[\frac{K_{21}-\beta}{\alpha-\beta}\right]e^{-\beta t}$$

$$Ct = \frac{D}{Vt}\left[\frac{K_{12}}{\beta-\alpha}\right]e^{-\alpha t} + \left[\frac{K_{12}}{\alpha-\beta}\right]e^{-\beta t}$$

where,

Cp = Drug concentration in plasma,

Ct = Drug concentration in tissue,

D = i.v. dose,

t = time after dose administration; α and β are distribution and elimination rate constants respectively.

The mathematical relationship of α and β to the rate constants are as below:

$$\alpha + \beta = K_{12} + K_{21} + K_2$$

$$\alpha.\beta = K_{21}.K_2$$

$$C_p = Ae^{-\alpha.t} + Be^{-\beta.t}$$

where A and B are intercepts on Y axis for distribution and elimination phase respectively. The values of A and B may be obtained graphically by the method of residuals.

Method of Residuals

This method is also known as feathering technique or peeling technique is an useful procedure for fitting a curve to the experimental data of a drug, which shows the necessity of a multi-compartment model.

For example, 1gm of cefgazolin was administered by rapid i.v. injection to a 12 kg healthy she goat. Blood samples were taken at different predetermined time intervals post drug administration and the each plasma sample was assayed for the drug. The following data were obtained.

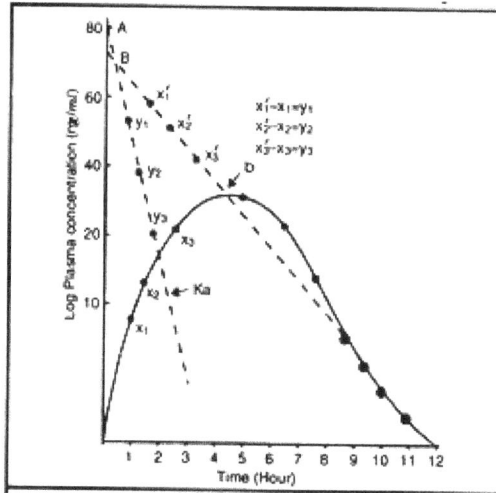

Showing Feathering technique for calculation of absorption rate constant (K_a)and elimination rate constant (β) after semilogarithmic plot of plasma concentration time profile of a drug.

Time (hr)	Plasma conc.(mg/ml)
0.25	43
0.50	32
1.	20
1.5	14

2.0	11
4.0	6.5
8.0	2.8
12.0	1.2
16.0	0.52

When this data will be plotted on semi-logarithmic graph paper, a curved line should be observed. The curved line relationship between the logarithm of the plasma concentration and time indicates that the drug is distributed in more than one compartment. From these data, a bi-exponential equation. may be derived by method of residuals.

From the bi-exponential curve it can be seen that the initial distribution rate is more rapid than the elimination rate. This explains that the rate constant α will be larger than rate constant β. Therefore, at some later time the term $Ae^{-\alpha.t}$ will approach zero while B will still have a value. At this time Equation $C_p = Ae^{-\alpha.t} + Be^{-\beta.t}$ will reduce to:

$$Cp = Be^{-\beta.t}$$

The rate constant β can be obtained from the slope (-β/2.3) of a straight line representing the terminal exponential phase. The $t_{1/2\beta}$ for the elimination phase can be derived from the following relationship.

$$t_1/2\beta = \frac{0.693}{\beta}$$

The new line obtained by graphing the logarithm of the residual plasma concentration (Cp − C'p) against time, represents the a phase,

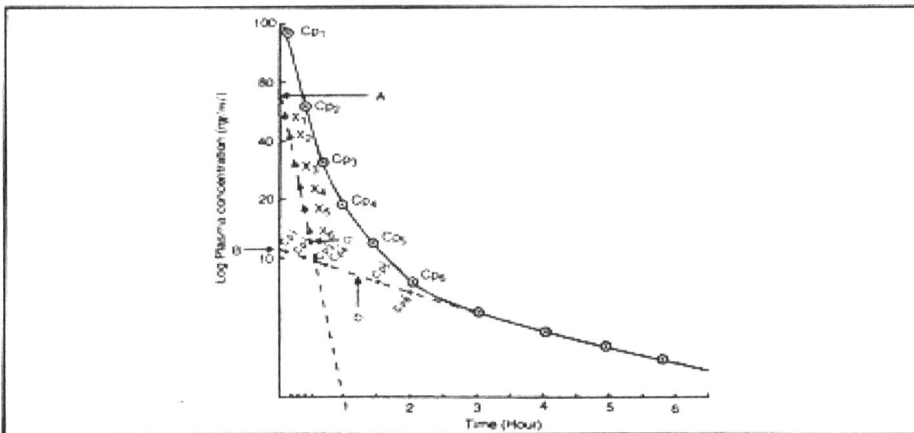

Sernllogulthmk plot of plasma concentnadons against Mae for a drug demonstrating first-order asomtlon and elimination kinetics, X_1, X_2, X_3, X_4, X_5 and X_6 has been calculated by method of residuals. (It is an Imaginary plot for a drug.)

Different pharmacokinetic parameters may be derived by proper substitution of rate constants α, β and intercepts A and B into the following equations:

$$K_2 = \frac{\alpha.\beta(A+B)}{A.\beta + B.\alpha}$$

$$K_{12} = \frac{A.B(\beta - \alpha)^2}{(A+B)(A.\beta + B.\alpha)}$$

$$K_{21} = \frac{A.\beta + B.\alpha}{A+B}$$

References

- S.K. Balani; V.S.Devishree; G.T. Miwa; L.S. Gan; J.T. Wu; F.W. Lee (2005). "Strategy of utilizing in vitro and in vivo ADME tools for lead optimization and drug candidate selection". Curr Top Med Chem. 5 (11): 1033–8. Doi:10.2174/156802605774297038. PMID 16181128

- Pharmacokinetic-models-concept-and-types, pharmacology-2: biologydiscussion.com, Retrieved 26 April, 2019

- Heaney, Robert P. (2001). "Factors Influencing the Measurement of Bioavailability, Taking Calcium as a Model". The Journal of Nutrition. 131 (4): 1344S–8S. doi:10.1093/jn/131.4.1344S. PMID 11285351

- Griffin, J. P. The Textbook of Pharmaceutical Medicine (6th ed.). Jersey: BMJ Books. ISBN 978-1-4051-8035-1

- Mizuno N, Niwa T, Yotsumoto Y, Sugiyama Y (September 2003). "Impact of drug transporter studies on drug discovery and development". Pharmacol. Rev. 55 (3): 425–61. doi:10.1124/pr.55.3.1. PMID 12869659

Pharmacodynamics

Pharmacodynamics refers to the study of the physiologic and biochemical effects of drugs. This chapter has been carefully written to provide an easy understanding of the varied facets of pharmacodynamics such as dose-response relationship, Schild regression and pharmacodynamics modeling.

Pharmacodynamics refers to the relationship between drug concentration at the site of action and the resulting effect, including the time course and intensity of therapeutic and adverse effects. The effect of a drug present at the site of action is determined by that drug's binding with a receptor. Receptors may be present on neurons in the central nervous system (i.e. opiate receptors) to depress pain sensation, on cardiac muscle to affect the intensity of contraction, or even within bacteria to disrupt maintenance of the bacterial cell wall.

For most drugs, the concentration at the site of the receptor determines the intensity of a drug's effect. However, other factors affect drug response as well. Density of receptors on the cell surface, the mechanism by which a signal is transmitted into the cell by second messengers (substances within the cell), or regulatory factors that control gene translation and protein production may influence drug effect. This multilevel regulation results in variation of sensitivity to drug effect from one individual to another and also determines enhancement of or tolerance to drug effects.

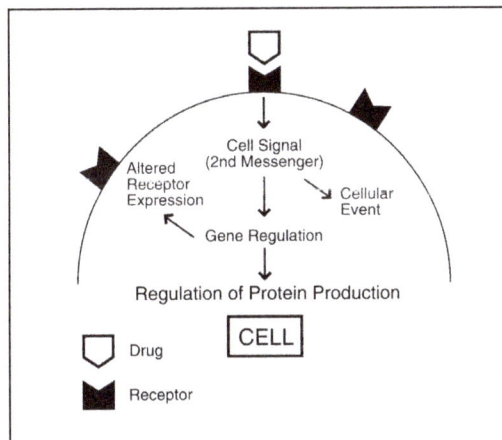

Relationship of drug concentration to drug effect at the receptor site.

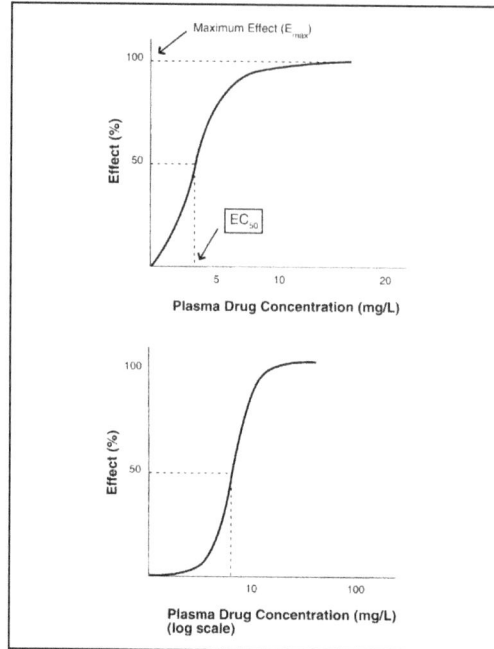

Relationship of drug concentration at the receptor site to effect (as a percentage of maximal effect).

In the simplest examples of drug effect, there is a relationship between the concentration of drug at the receptor site and the pharmacologic effect. If enough concentrations are tested, a maximum effect (E_{max}) can be determined . When the logarithm of concentration is plotted versus effect, one can see that there is a concentration below which no effect is observed and a concentration above which no greater effect is achieved.

One way of comparing drug potency is by the concentration at which 50% of the maximum effect is achieved. This is referred to as the 50% effective concentration or EC_{50}. When two drugs are tested in the same individual, the drug with a lower EC_{50} would be considered more potent. This means that a lesser amount of a more potent drug is needed to achieve the same effect as a less potent drug.

The EC_{50} does not, however, indicate other important determinants of drug response, such as the duration of effect. Duration of effect is determined by a complex set of factors, including the time that a drug is engaged on the receptor as well as intracellular signaling and gene regulation.

For some drugs, the effectiveness can decrease with continued use. This is referred to as tolerance. Tolerance may be caused by pharmacokinetic factors, such as increased drug metabolism, that decrease the concentrations achieved with a given dose. There can also be pharmacodynamic tolerance, which occurs when the same concentration at the receptor site results in a reduced effect with repeated exposure. An example of drug tolerance is the use of opiates in the management of chronic pain. It is not uncommon to find these patients requiring increased doses of the opiate over time. Tolerance can be described in terms of the dose– response curve, as shown in figure below.

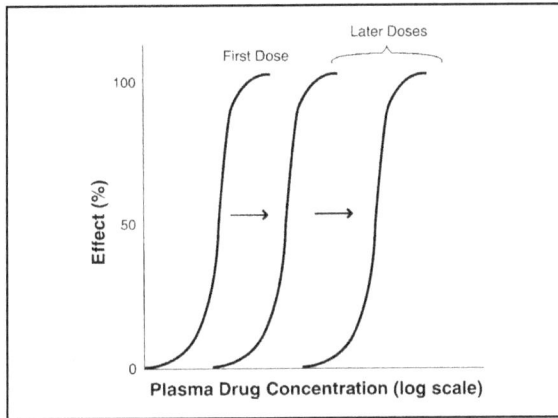

Demonstration of tolerance to drug effect with repeated dosing.

To assess the effect that a drug regimen is likely to have, the clinician should consider pharmacokinetic and pharmacodynamic factors. Both are important in determining a drug's effect.

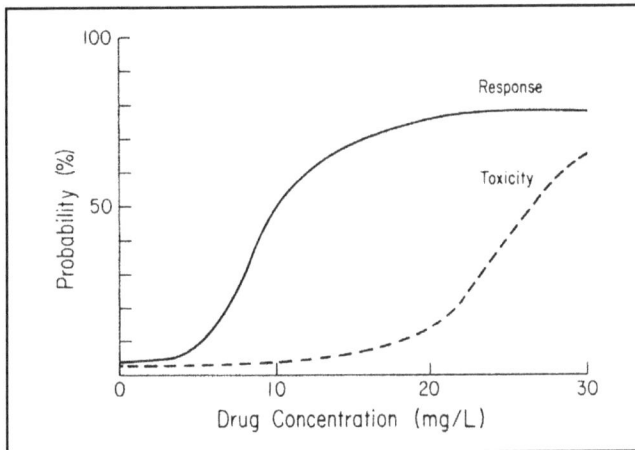

Relationship between drug concentration and drug effects for a hypothetical drug.

Therapeutic Drug Monitoring

Therapeutic drug monitoring is defined as the use of assay procedures for determination of drug concentrations in plasma, and the interpretation and application of the resulting concentration data to develop safe and effective drug regimens. If performed properly, this process allows for the achievement of therapeutic concentrations of a drug more rapidly and safely than can be attained with empiric dose changes. Together with observations of the drug's clinical effects, it should provide the safest approach to optimal drug therapy.

The usefulness of plasma drug concentration data is based on the concept that pharmacologic response is closely related to drug concentration at the site of action. For certain drugs, studies in patients have provided information on the plasma concentration range that is safe and effective in treating specific diseases—the therapeutic range. Within this therapeutic range, the desired effects of the drug are observed. Below it, there is greater probability that the therapeutic benefits are not realized; above it, toxic effects may occur.

No absolute boundaries divide subtherapeutic, therapeutic, and toxic drug concentrations. A gray area usually exists for most drugs in which these concentrations overlap due to variability in individual patient response. Numerous pharmacokinetic characteristics of a drug may result in variability in the plasma concentration achieved with a given dose when administered to various patients. This interpatient variability is primarily attributed to one or more of the following:

- Variations in drug absorption.

- Variations in drug distribution.

- Differences in an individual's ability to metabolize and eliminate the drug (e.g. genetics).

- Disease states (renal or hepatic insufficiency) or physiologic states (e.g. extremes of age, obesity) that alter drug absorption, distribution, or elimination.

- Drug interactions.

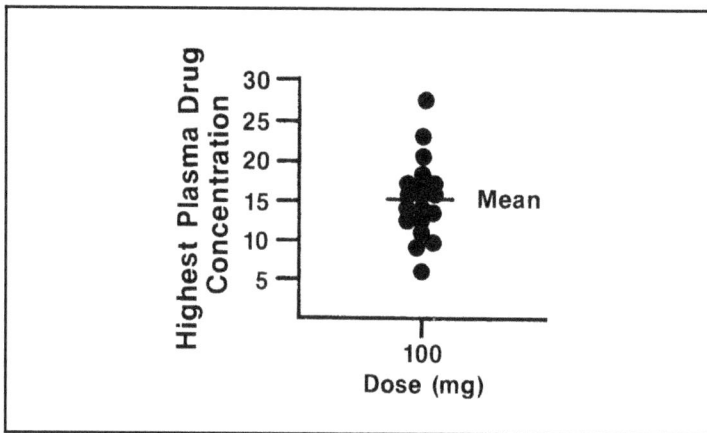

Example of variability in plasma drug concentration among subjects given the same drug dose.

Therapeutic monitoring using drug concentration data is valuable when:

- A good correlation exists between the pharmacologic response and plasma concentration. Over at least a limited concentration range, the intensity of pharmacologic effects should increase with plasma concentration. This relationship allows us to predict pharmacologic effects with changing plasma drug concentrations.

- Wide intersubject variation in plasma drug concentrations results from a given dose.

- The drug has a narrow therapeutic index (i.e. the therapeutic concentration is close to the toxic concentration).

- The drug's desired pharmacologic effects cannot be assessed readily by other simple means (e.g. blood pressure measurement for antihypertensives).

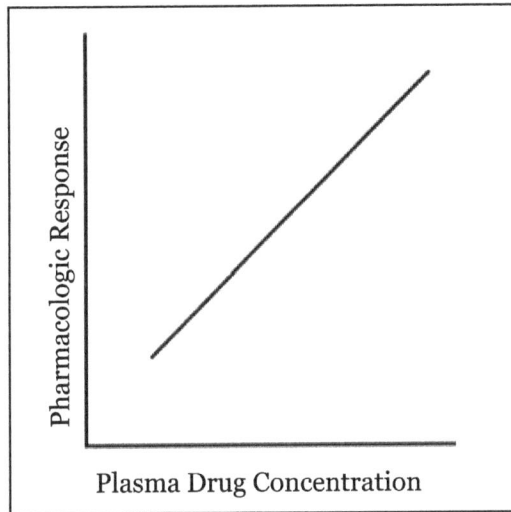

When pharmacologic effects relate to plasma drug concentrations,
he latter can be used to predict the former.

The value of therapeutic drug monitoring is limited in situations in which:

- There is no well-defined therapeutic plasma concentration range.

- The formation of pharmacologically active metabolites of a drug complicates the application of plasma drug concentration data to clinical effect unless metabolite concentrations are also considered.

- Toxic effects may occur at unexpectedly low drug concentrations as well as at high concentrations.

- There are no significant consequences associated with too high or too low levels.

Theophylline is an excellent example of a drug in which significant interpatient variability in pharmacokinetic properties exists. This is important from a clinical standpoint as subtle changes in serum concentrations may result in marked changes in drug response. Figure shows the relationship between theophylline concentration (x-axis, on a logarithmic scale) and its pharmacologic effect, (changes in pulmonary function [y-axis]). This figure illustrates that as the concentration of theophylline increases, so does the intensity of the response for some patients. Wide interpatient variability is also shown.

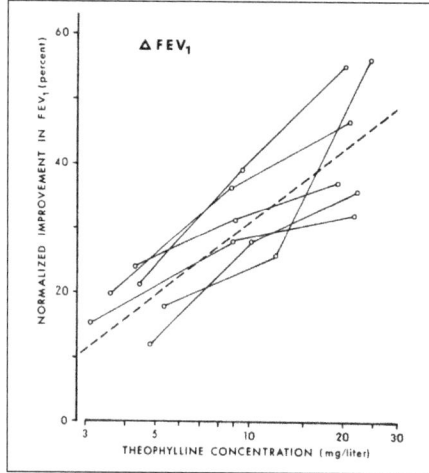

Relationship between plasma theophylline concentration and change
in forced expiratory volume (FEV) in asthmatic patients.

Figure outlines the process clinicians may choose to follow in making drug dosing decisions by using therapeutic drug monitoring. Figure shows the relationship of pharmacokinetic and pharmacodynamic factors.

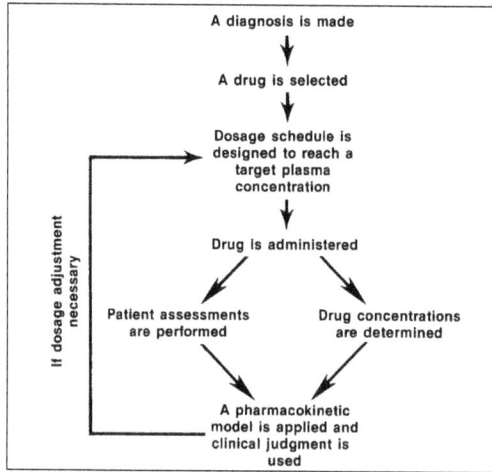

Process for reaching dosage decisions with therapeutic drug monitoring.

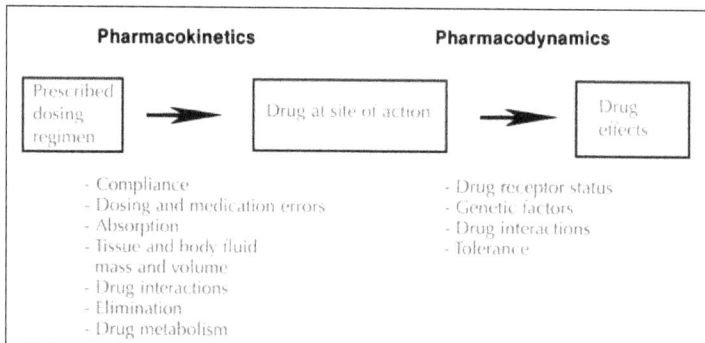

Relationship of pharmacokinetics and pharmacodynamics and factors that affect each.

DRUG ACTION AND PHARMACODYNAMICS

Drug action refers to the initial consequence of a drug-receptor interaction, and drug effect, which refers to the subsequent effects. The drug action of digoxin, for example, is inhibition of membrane Na^+/K^+-ATPase; the drug effect is augmentation of cardiac contractility. In this example, the clinical response might comprise improved exercise tolerance.

Not all drugs exert their pharmacologic actions via receptor-mediated mechanisms. The action of some drugs—including inhalation anesthetic agents, osmotic diuretics, purgatives, antiseptics, antacids, chelating agents, and urinary acidifying and alkalinizing agents—is attributed to their chemical action or physicochemical properties. Certain cancer and antiviral chemotherapeutic agents, which are analogues of pyrimidine and purine bases, elicit their effects when they are incorporated into nucleic acids and serve as substrates for DNA or RNA synthesis. The effect of most drugs, however, results from their interactions with receptors. These interactions and the resulting conformational changes in the receptor initiate biochemical and physiologic changes that characterize the drug's response.

Drug Concentration and Effect

Drug therapy is intended to result in a particular pharmacologic response of desired intensity and duration while avoiding adverse drug reactions. The relationship between the administered dose and the clinical response has been investigated for some drugs using a pharmacokinetic/pharmacodynamic (PK/PD) modeling approach, which is generally based on the plasma concentration-response relationship. For other drugs, a simpler relationship between the concentration and effect in an idealized in vitro system is modeled mathematically to conceptualize receptor occupancy and drug response. The model assumes that the drug interacts reversibly with its receptor and produces an effect proportional to the number of receptors occupied, up to a maximal effect when all receptors are occupied. The reaction scheme for the model is:

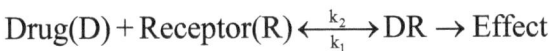

$$\text{Drug(D)} + \text{Receptor(R)} \underset{k_1}{\overset{k_2}{\longleftrightarrow}} \text{DR} \rightarrow \text{Effect}$$

in which k_2 and k_1 are rate constants.

The relationship between effect and the concentration of free drug for the model is given by the Hill equation, which can be written as:

$$E = \frac{E_{max} \times C_n}{EC_{50} + C_n}$$

in which E is the effect observed at concentration C, E_{max} is the maximal response that can be produced by the drug (efficacy), EC_{50} is the concentration of drug that produces

50% of maximal effect (potency), and the Hill coefficient n is the slope of the $\log_{10}$ concentration-effect relationship (sensitivity).

The above equation describes a rectangular hyperbola when response (y-axis) is plotted against concentration (x-axis). However, dose- or concentration-response data is generally plotted as drug effect (y-axis) against $\log_{10}$ dose or concentration (x-axis). The transformation yields a sigmoidal curve that allows the potency of different drugs to be readily compared. In addition, the effect of drugs used at therapeutic concentrations commonly falls on the portion of the sigmoidal curve that is approximately linear, ie, between 20% and 80% of maximal effect. This makes for easier interpretation of the plotted data.

Agonists and Antagonists

An agonist is a drug that binds to receptors and thereby alters (stabilizes) the proportion of receptors in the active conformation, resulting in a biologic response. A full agonist results in a maximal response by occupying all or a fraction of receptors. A partial agonist results in less than a maximal response even when the drug occupies all of the receptors.

There are four types of drug antagonism. Chemical antagonism involves chemical interaction between a drug and either a chemical or another drug leading to a reduced or nil response. Physiologic antagonism occurs when two drugs acting on different receptors and pathways exert opposing actions on the same physiologic system. Pharmacokinetic antagonism is the result of one drug suppressing the effect of a second drug by reducing its absorption, altering its distribution, or increasing its rate of elimination. Pharmacologic antagonism occurs when the antagonist inhibits the effect of a full or partial agonist by acting on the same pathway but not necessarily on the same receptor.

Pharmacologic antagonists comprise three subcategories. A reversible competitive antagonist results in inhibition that can be overcome by increasing the concentration of agonist. The presence of a reversible competitive antagonist causes a parallel rightward shift of the log concentration-effect curve of the agonist without altering E_{max} or EC_{50}. An irreversible competitive antagonist also involves competition between agonist and antagonist for the same receptors, but stronger binding forces prevent the effect of the antagonist being fully reversed, even at high agonist concentrations. The presence of an irreversible competitive antagonist causes a rightward shift of the log concentration-effect curve of the agonist that generally displays decreased slope and reduced maximum effect. A noncompetitive antagonist inhibits agonist activity by blocking one of the sequential reactions between receptor activation and the pharmacologic response. Noncompetitive antagonism is generally reversible but can be irreversible. Noncompetitive antagonists and irreversible competitive antagonists cause similar perturbations in the log concentration-effect curve of agonists. Isolated tissue experiments are used to distinguish the two subcategories, because noncompetitive antagonists are generally reversible.

Agonists, but not antagonists, elicit an effect even when they bind to the same site on the same receptor. An explanation is provided by both structural and functional studies, which indicate that receptors exist in at least two conformations, active and inactive, and these are in equilibrium. Because agonists have a higher affinity for the receptor's active conformation, agonists drive the equilibrium to the active state, thereby activating the receptor. Conversely, antagonists have a higher affinity for the receptor's inactive conformation and push the equilibrium to the inactive state, producing no effect.

The concept of spare receptors explains a maximum response being achieved when only a fraction of the total number of receptors is occupied. For example, an action potential and maximal twitch of muscle fibers is elicited when 0.13% of the total number of receptors at a skeletal neuromuscular junction is simultaneously activated. From a functional perspective, spare receptors are significant, because they increase both the sensitivity and speed of a tissue's responsiveness to a ligand.

Structure-activity Relationships

Structure-activity relationships are exploited in drug design, because small changes in chemical structure can produce profound changes in potency. For example, the substitution of a proton by a methyl group accounts for codeine being ~1,000 times less potent than morphine in its action on opioid receptors.

Signal Transduction and Drug Action

Most receptors are proteins. The best characterized of these are regulatory proteins, enzymes, transport proteins, and structural proteins. Nucleic acids are also important drug receptors, particularly for cancer chemotherapeutic agents.

The receptors for several neurotransmitters modulate the opening and closing of ion channels through ligand gating or voltage gating. The nicotinic acetylcholine receptor is an example of a ligand-gated receptor; it allows Na^+ to flow down its concentration gradient into cells, resulting in depolarization. Most clinically useful neuromuscular blocking drugs compete with acetylcholine for the receptor but do not initiate ion-channel opening. Other ligand-gated ion channels include the CNS receptors for the excitatory amino acids (glutamate and aspartate), the inhibitory amino acids (γ-aminobutyric acid [GABA] and glycine), and certain serotonin (5-HT3) receptors. The sodium channel receptor is an example of a voltage-gated receptor; these are present in the membranes of excitable nerve, cardiac, and skeletal muscle cells. In the resting state, the Na^+/K^+-ATPase pump in these cells maintains an intracellular Na^+ concentration much lower than that in the extracellular environment. Membrane depolarization causes channel opening and a transient influx of Na^+ ions, followed by inactivation and return to the resting state. The action of local anesthetics is due to their direct interaction with voltage-gated Na^+ channels.

Many transmembrane receptors are linked to guanosine triphosphate binding proteins, which activate second messenger systems. Two important second messenger systems are cyclic adenosine monophosphate (cAMP) and the phosphoinositides. In cAMP second messenger systems, binding of the ligand to the receptor increases or decreases adenylyl cyclase activity, which in turn regulates the formation of cAMP from adenosine triphosphate. The activation of protein kinase A by cAMP results in the phosphorylation of proteins and a physiologic effect. From a therapeutic standpoint, drug binding to β-adrenergic, histamine H_2, or dopamine D_1 receptors activates adenylyl cyclase, whereas binding to muscarinic M_2, α_2-adrenergic, dopamine D_2, opiate μ and δ, adenosine A_1, or GABA type B receptors inhibits adenylyl cyclase. In phosphoinositide second messenger systems, membrane phosphatidylinositol 4,5-biphosphate is hydrolyzed to 1,4,5-trisphosphate (IP3) and 1,2-diacylglycerol (DAG) by activation of phospholipase C. Both IP3 and DAG activate kinases, and in the case of IP3, this involves the mobilization of calcium from intracellular stores. The action of numerous drugs is due to their interaction with receptors that rely on these second messengers, which include α_1-adrenergic, muscarinic M_1 or M_2, serotonin 5-HT2, and thyrotropin-releasing hormone receptors.

Protein tyrosine kinase receptors are generally transmembrane enzymes that phosphorylate proteins exclusively on tyrosine residues, rather than on serine or threonine residues. They include endocrine hormone receptors for insulin and receptors for several growth hormones.

Intracellular receptors mediate the action of hormones such as glucocorticoids, estrogen, and thyroid hormone and related drugs. The hormones, which regulate gene expression in the nucleus, are lipophilic and freely diffuse through the cell membrane to reach the receptor. Glucocorticoid receptors reside predominantly in the cytoplasm in an inactive form until they bind to the glucocorticoid steroid ligand. This results in receptor activation and translocation to the nucleus, where the receptor interacts with specific DNA sequences. Unlike glucocorticoid receptors, the receptors for estrogen and thyroid hormone reside in the nucleus.

Intracellular receptors are also important in mediating the action of antimicrobial drugs, including the penicillins, sulfonamides, trimethoprim, aminoglycosides, phenicols, macrolides, and fluoroquinolones. The mechanisms of action include inhibition of bacterial protein synthesis, inhibition of cell wall synthesis, inhibition of enzymatic activity, alteration of cell membrane permeability, and blockade of specific biochemical pathways.

Receptor-mediated mechanisms of action of several classes of anthelmintics are well understood. For example, the benzimidazoles and pro-benzimidazoles bind to nematode tubulin, preventing its polymerization during microtubular assembly and thus disrupting cell division. Depletion of ATP as the result of salicylanilides uncoupling oxidative phosphorylation and the inhibition of enzymes in the glycolytic pathway by benzene sulfonamides are other examples. Several classes of anthelmintics interfere with neurotransmission in parasites. A case in point is macrocyclic lactones, which potentiate inhibitory neurotransmission via GABA and glutamate-gated chlorine channels.

Drug Dose and Clinical Response

To make rational therapeutic decisions, it is necessary to understand the fundamental concepts linking drug doses to concentrations to clinical responses. The concentration-response relationships for drugs may be graded or quantal. A graded concentration-response curve can be constructed for responses measured on a continuous scale, eg, heart rate. Graded concentration-response curves relate the intensity of response to the size of the dose and, hence, are useful to characterize the actions of drugs. A quantal concentration-response curve can be constructed for drugs that elicit an all-or-none response, eg, presence or absence of convulsions. For most drugs, the doses required to produce a specified quantal effect in a population are log normally distributed, so that the frequency distribution of responses plotted against log dose is a gaussian normal distribution curve. The percentage of the population requiring a particular dose to exhibit the effect can be determined from this curve. When these data are plotted as a cumulative frequency distribution, a sigmoidal dose-response curve is generated.

The equilibrium dissociation constant of the receptor-drug complex, K_D, is the ratio of rate constants for the reverse (k_2) and forward (k_1) reaction between the drug and receptor and the drug-receptor complex. K_D is also the drug concentration at which receptor occupancy is half of maximum. Drugs with a high K_D (low affinity) dissociate rapidly from receptors; conversely, drugs with a low K_D (high affinity) dissociate slowly from receptors. These effects impact the rate at which biologic responses end.

Potency refers to the concentration (EC_{50}) or dose (ED_{50}) of a drug required to produce 50% of the drug's maximal effect as depicted by a graded dose-response curve. EC_{50} equals K_D when there is a linear relationship between occupancy and response. Often, signal amplification occurs between receptor occupancy and response, which results in the EC_{50} for response being much less (ie, positioned to the left on the x-axis of the log dose-response curve) than K_D for receptor occupancy. Potency depends on both the affinity of a drug for its receptor and the efficiency with which drug-receptor interaction is coupled to response. The dose of drug required to produce an effect is inversely related to potency. In general, low potency is important only if it results in a need to administer the drug in large doses that are impractical. Quantal dose-response curves provide information on the potency of drugs that is different from the information derived from graded dose-response curves. In a quantal dose-response relationship, the ED_{50} is the dose at which 50% of individuals exhibit the specified quantal effect.

The median inhibitory concentration, or IC_{50}, is the concentration of an antagonist that reduces a specified response to 50% of the maximal possible effect.

Efficacy (also referred to as intrinsic activity) of a drug is the ability of the drug to elicit a response when it binds to the receptor. As discussed above, conformational changes in receptors as a result of drug occupancy initiate biochemical and physiologic events that characterize the drug's response. In some tissues, agonists demonstrating high efficacy can result in a maximal effect, even when only a small fraction of the receptors is occupied.

Selectivity refers to a drug's ability to preferentially produce a particular effect and is related to the structural specificity of drug binding to receptors. For example, cyclooxygenase-2 (COX-2) preferential NSAIDs demonstrate partial specificity for COX-2, the inducible enzyme formed at sites of inflammation. By comparison, COX-2 selective NSAIDs are without significant effect on COX-1, the constitutive enzyme that performs a range of physiologic functions. For certain drugs, selectivity is species dependent. For example, $S(+)$-carprofen is COX-2 selective in dogs and cats, nonselective of COX-1 and COX-2 in horses, and COX-2 preferential in calves.

Specificity of drug action relates to the number of different mechanisms involved. Examples of specific drugs include atropine (a muscarinic receptor antagonist), salbutamol (a β_2-adrenoceptor agonist), and cimetidine (an H_2- receptor antagonist). By contrast, nonspecific drugs result in drug effects through several mechanisms of action. For example, phenothiazine causes blockade of D_2-dopamine receptors, α-adrenergic receptors, and muscarinic receptors.

The affinity of a drug for a receptor describes how avidly the drug binds to the receptor (ie, the K_D). The chemical forces in drug-receptor interactions include electrostatic forces, van der Waal forces, and the forces associated with hydrogen bonds and hydrophobic bonds. Variation in the strength of these forces, and therefore the thermal energy in the system, determines the degree of association and dissociation of the drug and the receptor. Covalent binding of drug to receptor (exemplified by fluoroquinolones acting on bacteria) leads to formation of an irreversible link.

The therapeutic index of a drug is the ratio of the dose that results in an undesired effect to the dose that results in a desired effect. The therapeutic index of a drug is usually defined as the ratio of LD_{50} to ED_{50} (median lethal and median effective doses, respectively, in 50% of individuals), which indicates how selective the drug is in eliciting its desired effect. Values of LD_{50} and ED_{50} for this purpose are derived from quantal dose-response curves generated in animal studies.

The information obtained from dose- and concentration-response curves is critically important when choosing between drugs and when determining the dose to administer. A drug is chosen largely on the basis of its clinical effectiveness for a particular therapeutic indication. In this context, the drug concentration at the receptor (determined by the pharmacokinetic properties of the drug) and the efficacy of the drug-receptor complex are the primary determinants of a drug's clinical effectiveness. The administered dose of a drug, by comparison, depends to a greater extent on potency than on maximal efficacy.

The maximal efficacy of the drug-receptor complex to result in a graded effect is E_{max} or I_{max} on a graded dose-response curve. E_{max} or I_{max} is derived from a quantitative dose-response relationship for a single animal and varies among individuals. The extrapolation of this value of E_{max} to a clinical case is only an estimate, but it facilitates a comparison of the maximal efficacy of drugs that result in a specified effect by identical receptors. A drug's potency (ie, EC_{50}, ED_{50}, or IC_{50}) obtained from either graded or quantal dose-response curves is used to determine the dose that should be administered. The slope of the graded dose-response curve (n in the Hill equation, above) provides information concerning the dose range over which a drug elicits its effect. Other information concerning the selectivity of drug action and the therapeutic index is also obtained from the graded dose-response curve. When quantal effects are being considered, information concerning pharmacologic potency, selectivity of drug action, the margin of safety, and the potential variability of responsiveness among individuals is obtained from quantal dose-response curves.

Pharmacodynamics of Antimicrobial Drugs

The approach used to investigate the pharmacodynamics of antimicrobial drugs (and parasiticides) differs from that of other veterinary drugs on account of the need to address target pathogens that have structure, biochemistry, and capacity for replication which are markedly dissimilar to those of their mammalian host. The individual drugs within each group of antimicrobial drugs differ in potency and in antimicrobial spectrum of activity. The minimum inhibitory concentration (MIC), which is the lowest concentration of drug that completely inhibits bacterial growth, is determined in vitro as a measure of susceptibility of bacterial species and strains to a given drug. Importantly, the MIC_{50} provides a measure of potency, EC_{50}.

Other surrogate markers of bacteriologic effect exist and include the minimum bactericidal concentration (MBC), which is the concentration of antimicrobial drug that produces a 3-log-unit or 99.9% reduction in bacterial count, postantibiotic effect, sub-MIC postantibiotic effect, and time-kill data. More recently, the application of PK/PD principles to antimicrobial drug action has led to PK/PD integration and PK/PD modeling. PK/PD integration brings together data from PK and PD studies. The surrogate PK/PD index that best correlates with efficacy for a given drug is selected based on the drug's killing mechanism, namely concentration dependent, time dependent, or codependent (ie, both time and concentration determine outcome). The PK/PD index selected for aminogylycosides, which act by concentration-dependent killing mechanisms, is C_{max}/MIC ratio (C_{max} is the maximum plasma concentration after administration of a drug by a nonvascular route); for β-lactams, which act by time-dependent killing mechanisms, it is T>MIC (T is the time for which plasma concentration exceeds MIC, expressed as a percentage of the dosage interval); and for fluoroquinolones, which act by concentration-dependent killing mechanisms, AUC/MIC ratio (AUC is the area under the plasma drug concentration-time curve) is selected. The objective of PK/PD modeling is to define the three key pharmacodynamic properties that define any drug, namely E_{max} or I_{max} (efficacy); EC_{50} (or EC_{80} or EC_{90}) (potency); and slope (n) in the Hill equation, which indicates sensitivity and selectivity. PK/PD modeling permits breakpoint values to achieve a bacteriostatic or bactericidal effect, or bacterial eradication to be computed, which are used to optimize efficacy and minimize resistance.

Time-effect Relationships

The ability of drugs to reach the receptor is determined by pharmacokinetic parameters that characterize the absorption, distribution, and clearance of a drug. There may not be a simple temporal correlation between plasma concentration of a drug and its therapeutic effect. Plotting plasma concentrations (x-axis) versus therapeutic effect (y-axis) in chronologic order displays the data as a loop for some drugs. This phenomenon is referred to as hysteresis in the concentration-effect relationship. The effect of most drugs lag behind the plasma concentration. This results in a counterclockwise hysteresis loop. For example, the NSAID robenicoxib has prolonged local effects after blood concentrations have decreased below effective levels. A clockwise hysteresis loop is observed for cocaine and pseudoephedrine when tachyphylaxis develops. The temporal correlation between plasma concentration and therapeutic effect also varies for the different classes of antagonists. For instance, the extent and duration of action of a competitive antagonist depends on its concentration in plasma, which depends (in part) on its rate of elimination. This requires that the dose be adjusted accordingly to maintain plasma concentrations in the therapeutic range. By contrast, the duration of action of an irreversible antagonist is relatively independent of its rate of elimination and, therefore, plasma concentration, and more dependent on the rate of turnover of receptor molecules.

Down-regulation and Up-regulation of Receptors

The density of most receptors is not constant with time, which has important therapeutic implications. Down-regulation of receptors may occur as a result of continual stimulation by an agonist and manifests as the development of tachyphylaxis, which demonstrates a clockwise hysteresis loop in the concentration-effect relationship. Conversely, additional receptors can be synthesized in response to chronic receptor antagonism—a phenomenon known as up-regulation. Because more receptors are now available, a hyperreactive response occurs when the cell is exposed to an agonist.

TOXICODYNAMICS

Toxicodynamics, termed pharmacodynamics in pharmacology, describes the dynamic interactions of a toxicant with a biological target and its biological effects. A biological target, also known as the site of action, can be binding proteins, ion channels, DNA, or a variety of other receptors. When a toxicant enters an organism, it can interact with these receptors and produce structural or functional alterations. The mechanism of action of the toxicant, as determined by a toxicant's chemical properties, will determine what receptors are targeted and the overall toxic effect at the cellular level and organismal level.

Toxicants have been grouped together according to their chemical properties by way of quantitative structure-activity relationships (QSARs), which allows prediction of toxic action based on these properties. endocrine disrupting chemicals (EDCs) and carcinogens are examples of classes of toxicants that can act as QSARs. EDCs mimic or block transcriptional activation normally caused by natural steroid hormones. These types of chemicals can act on androgen receptors, estrogen receptors and thyroid hormone receptors. This mechanism can include such toxicants as dichlorodiphenyltrichloroethane (DDE) and polychlorinated biphenyls (PCBs). Another class of chemicals, carcinogens, are substances that cause cancer and can be classified as genotoxic or nongenotoxic carcinogens. These categories include toxicants such as polycyclic aromatic hydrocarbon (PAHs) and carbon tetrachloride (CCl_4).

The process of toxicodynamics can be useful for application in environmental risk assessment by implementing toxicokinetic-toxicodynamic (TKTD) models. TKTD models include phenomenas such as time-varying exposure, carry-over toxicity, organism recovery time, effects of mixtures, and extrapolation to untested chemicals and species. Due to their advantages, these types of models may be more applicable for risk assessment than traditional modeling approaches.

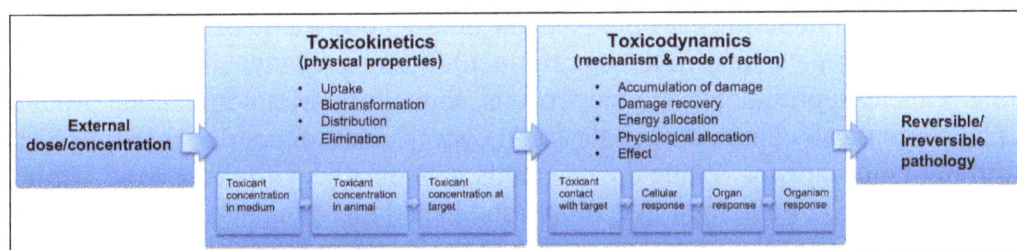

A box model explaining the processes of toxicokinetics and toxicodynamics.

While toxicokinetics describes the changes in the concentrations of a toxicant over time due to the uptake, biotransformation, distribution and elimination of toxicants, toxicodynamics involves the interactions of a toxicant with a biological target and the functional or structural alterations in a cell that can eventually lead to a toxic effect. Depending on the toxicant's chemical reactivity and vicinity, the toxicant may be able to interact with the biological target. Interactions between a toxicant and the biological target may also be more specific, where high-affinity binding sites increase the selectivity of interactions. For this reason, toxicity may be expressed primarily in certain tissues or organs. The targets are often receptors on the cell surface or in the cytoplasm and nucleus. Toxicants can either induce an unnecessary response or inhibit a natural response, which can cause damage. If the biological target is critical and the damage is severe enough, irreversible injury can occur first at the molecular level, which will translate into effects at higher levels of organization.

Endocrine Disruptors

EDCs are generally considered to be toxicants that either mimic or block the transcriptional activation normally caused by natural steroid hormones. These chemicals include those acting on androgen receptors, estrogen receptors and thyroid hormone receptors.

Effects of Endocrine Disruptors

Endocrine disrupting chemicals can interfere with the endocrine system in a number of ways including hormone synthesis, storage/release, transport and clearance, receptor recognition and binding, and postreceptor activation.

In wildlife, exposure to EDCs can result in altered fertility, reduced viability of offspring, impaired hormone secretion or activity and modified reproductive anatomy. The reproductive anatomy of offspring can particularly be affected if maternal exposure occurs. In females, this includes mammary glands, fallopian tubes, uterus, cervix, and vagina. In males, this includes the prostate, seminal vesicles, epididymitis and testes. Exposure of fish to EDCs has also been associated with abnormal thyroid function, decreased fertility, decreased hatching success, de-feminization and masculinization of female fish and alteration of immune function.

Endocrine disruption as a mode of action for xenobiotics was brought into awareness by Theo Colborn. Endocrine disrupting chemicals are known to accumulate in body tissue and are highly persistent in the environment. Many toxicants are known EDCs including pesticides, phthalates, phytoestrogens, some industrial/commercial products, and pharmaceuticals. These chemicals are known to cause endocrine disruption via a few different mechanisms. While the mechanism associated with the thyroid hormone receptor is not well understood, two more established mechanisms involve the inhibition of the androgen receptor and activation of the estrogen receptor.

Androgen Receptor Mediated

Certain toxicants act as endocrine disruptors by interacting with the androgen receptor. DDE is one example of a chemical that acts via this mechanism. DDE is a metabolite of DDT that is widespread in the environment. Although production of DDT has been banned in the Western world, this chemical is extremely persistent and is still commonly found in the environment along with its metabolite DDE. DDE is an antiandrogen, which means it alters the expression of specific androgen-regulated genes, and is an androgen receptor (AR)-mediated mechanism. DDE is a lipophilic compound which diffuses into the cell and binds to the AR. Through binding, the receptor is inactivated and cannot bind to the androgen response element on DNA. This inhibits the transcription of androgen-responsive genes which can have serious consequences for exposed wildlife. In 1980, there was a spill in Lake Apopka, Florida which released the pesticide dicofol and DDT along with its metabolites. The neonatal and juvenile alligators present in this lake have been extensively studied and observed to have altered plasma hormone concentrations, decreased clutch viability, increased juvenile mortality, and morphological abnormalities in the testis and ovary.

Estrogen Receptor Mediated

Toxicants may also cause endocrine disruption through interacting with the estrogen receptor. This mechanism has been well-studied with PCBs. These chemicals have been used as coolants and lubricants in transformers and other electrical equipment due to their insulating properties. A purely anthropogenic substance, PCBs are no longer in production in the United States due to the adverse health effects associated with exposure, but they are highly persistent and are still widespread in the environment. PCBs are a xenoestrogen, which elicit an enhancing (rather than inhibiting) response, and are mediated by the estrogen receptor. These are often referred to as estrogen mimics because they mimic the effects of estrogen. PCBs often build up in sediments and bioaccumulate in organisms. These chemicals diffuse into the nucleus and bind to the estrogen receptor. The estrogen receptor is kept in an inactive conformation through interactions with proteins such as heat shock proteins 59, 70, and 90. After the toxicant binding occurs, the estrogen receptor is activated and forms a homodimer complex which seeks out estrogen response elements in the DNA. The binding of the complex to these elements causes a rearrangement of the chromatin and transcription of the gene, resulting in production of a specific protein. In doing this, PCBs elicit an estrogenic response which can affect numerous functions within the organism. These effects are observed in various aquatic species. The levels of PCBs in marine mammals are often very high as a result of bioaccumulation. Studies have demonstrated that PCBs are responsible for reproductive impairment in the harbor seal (*Phoca vitulina*). Similar effects have been found in the grey seal (*Halichoerus grypus*), the ringed seal (*Pusa hispida*) and the California sea lion (*Zalophys californinus*). In the grey seals and ringed seals, uterine occlusions and stenosis were found which led to sterility. If exposed to a xenoestrogen such as PCBs, male fish have also been seen to produce vitellogenin. Vitellogenin is an egg protein female fish normally produce but is not usually present in males except at very low concentrations. This is often used as a biomarker for EDCs.

Carcinogens

Carcinogens are defined as any substance that causes cancer. The toxicodynamics of carcinogens can be complex due to the varying mechanisms of action for different carcinogenic toxicants. Because of their complex nature, carcinogens are classified as either genotoxic or nongenotoxic carcinogens.

Effects of Carcinogens

The effects of carcinogens are most often related to human exposures but mammals are not the only species that can be affected by cancer-causing toxicants. Many studies have shown that cancer can develop in fish species as well. Neoplasms occurring in epithelial tissue such as the liver, gastrointestinal tract, and the pancreas have been linked to various environmental toxicants. Carcinogens preferentially target the liver in fish and develop hepatocellular and biliary lesions.

Genotoxic Carcinogens

Genotoxic carcinogens interact directly with DNA and genetic material or indirectly by their reactive metabolites. Toxicants such as PAHs can be genotoxic carcinogens to aquatic organisms. PAHs are widely spread throughout the environment through the incomplete burning of coal, wood, or petroleum products. Although PAHs do not bioaccumulate in vertebrate tissue, many studies have confirmed that certain PAH compounds such as benzo(a)pyrene, benz(a)anthracene, and Benzofluoranthene, are bioavailable and responsible for liver diseases like cancer in wild fish populations. One mechanism of action for genotoxic carcinogens includes the formation of DNA adducts. Once the PAH compound enters an organism, it becomes metabolized and available for biotransformation.

The biotransformation process can activate the PAH compound and transform it into a diol epoxide, which is a very reactive intermediate. These diol-epoxides covalently bind with DNA base pairs, most often with guanine and adenine to form stable adducts within the DNA structure. The binding of diol epoxides and DNA base pairs blocks polymerase replication activity. This blockage ultimately contributes to an increase in DNA damage by reducing repair activity.

Due to these processes, PAH compounds are thought to play a role in the initiation and early promotion stage of carcinogenesis. Fish exposed to PAHs develop a range of liver lesions, some of which are characteristic of hepatocarcinogenicity.

Nongenotoxic Carcinogens

Nongenotoxic, or epigenetic carcinogens are different and slightly more ambiguous than genotoxic carcinogens since they are not directly carcinogenic. Nongenotoxic carcinogens act by secondary mechanisms that do not directly damage genes. This type of carcinogenesis does not change the sequence of DNA; instead it alters the expression or repression of certain genes by a wide variety of cellular processes. Since these toxicants do not directly act on DNA, little is known about the mechanistic pathway. It has been proposed that modification of gene expression from nongenotoxic carcinogens can occur by oxidative stress, peroxisome proliferation, suppression of apoptosis, alteration of intercellular communication, and modulation of metabolizing enzymes.

Carbon tetrachloride is an example of a probable nongenotoxic carcinogen to aquatic vertebrates. Historically, carbon tetrachloride has been used in pharmaceutical production, petroleum refining, and as an industrial solvent. Due to its widespread industrial use and release into the environment, carbon tetrachloride has been found in drinking water and therefore, has become a concern for aquatic organisms. Because of its high hepatotoxic properties, carbon tetrachloride could potentially be linked to liver cancer. Experimental cancer studies have shown that carbon tetrachloride may cause benign and malignant liver tumors to rainbow trout. carbon tetrachloride works as a nongenotoxic carcinogen by formulating free radicals which induce oxidative stress. It has been proposed that once carbon tetrachloride enters the organism, it is metabolized to trichloromethyl and trichloromethyl peroxy radicals by the CYP2E1 enzyme. The more reactive radical, trichloromethyl peroxy, can attack polyunsaturated fatty acids in the cellular membrane to form fatty acid free radicals and initiate lipid peroxidation. The attack on the cellular membrane increases its permeability, causing a leakage of enzymes and disrupts cellular calcium homeostasis. This loss of calcium homeostasis activates calcium dependent degradative enzymes and cytotoxicity, causing hepatic damage. The regenerative and proliferative changes that occur in the liver during this time could increase the frequency of genetic damage, resulting in a possible increase of cancer.

Applications

Toxicodynamics can be used in combination with toxicokinetics in environmental risk assessment to determine the potential effects of releasing a toxicant into the environment. The most widely used method of incorporating this are TKTD models.

Setup of TKTD Models

Both toxicokinetics and toxicodynamics have now been described, and using these definitions models were formed, where the internal concentration (TK) and damage (TD) are simulated in response to exposure. TK and TD are separated in the model to allow for the identification of properties of toxicants that determine TK and those that determine TD. To use this type of model, parameter values for TK processes need to be obtained first. Second, the TD parameters need to be estimated. Both of these steps require a large database of toxicity information for parameterization. After establishing all the parameter values for the TKTD model, and using basic scientific precautions, the model can be used to predict toxic effects, calculate recovery times for organisms, or establish extrapolations from the model to toxicity of untested toxicants and species.

It has been argued that the current challenges facing risk assessments can be addressed with TKTD modeling. TKTD models were derived in response to a couple of factors. One is the lack of time being considered as a factor in toxicity and risk assessment. Some of the earliest developed TKTD models, such as the Critical Body

Residue (CBR) model and Critical Target Occupation (CTO) model, have considered time as a factor but a criticism has been that they are for very specific circumstances such as reversibly acting toxicants or irreversibly acting toxicants. Further extrapolation of the CTO and CBR models are DEBtox, which can model sublethal endpoints, and hazard versions of the CTO, which takes into account stochastic death as opposed to individual tolerance. Another significant step to developing TKTD models was the incorporation of a state variable for damage. By using damage as a toxicodynamic state-variable, modeling intermediate recovery rates can be accomplished for toxicants that act reversibly with their targets, without the assumptions of instant recovery (CBR model) or irreversible interactions (CTO model). TKTD models that incorporate damage are the Damage Assessment Model (DAM) and the Threshold Damage Model (TDM). For what may seem like straightforward endpoints, a variety of different TKTD approaches exist. A review of the assumptions and hypotheses of each was previously published in the creation of a general unified threshold model of survival (GUTS).

Advantages for Risk Assessment

As referenced above, TKTD models have several advantages to traditional models for risk assessments. The principal advantages to using TKTD models are:

- The consequences of time-varying or repeated exposures can be explained and simulated by the TKTD model.

- Carry-over toxicity as well as delayed effects can be simulated, whether the carry-over toxicity is due to TK or TD or both. In this way, TKTD models can quantify risks from pulsed or fluctuating exposures.

- Organism recovery time depends on the time course of TK and TD, which makes the TKTD models suitable for calculating organism recovery time.

- TKTD models have the potential to predict effects of mixtures and also be used as mechanism-based extrapolation to untested toxicants or untested species.

- Linking TKTD models with Individual Based Models (IBM) may improve risk assessment of toxicants by simulating temporal aspects as well as ecological aspects.

Due to its advantages, TKTD models may be more powerful than the traditional dose-response models because of their incorporation of chemical concentrations as well as temporal dimensions. Toxicodynamic modeling (such as TKTD models) has been shown to be a useful tool for toxicological research, with increasing opportunities to use these results in risk assessment to permit a more scientifically based risk assessment that is less reliable on animal testing. Overall, these types of models can formalize knowledge about the toxicity of toxicants and organism sensitivity, create new hypotheses, and simulate temporal aspects of toxicity, making them useful tools for risk assessment.

DOSE–RESPONSE RELATIONSHIP

The dose–response relationship, or exposure–response relationship, describes the magnitude of the response of an organism, as a function of exposure (or doses) to a stimulus or stressor (usually a chemical) after a certain exposure time. Dose–response relationships can be described by dose–response curves. A stimulus response function or stimulus response curve is defined more broadly as the response from any type of stimulus, not limited to chemicals.

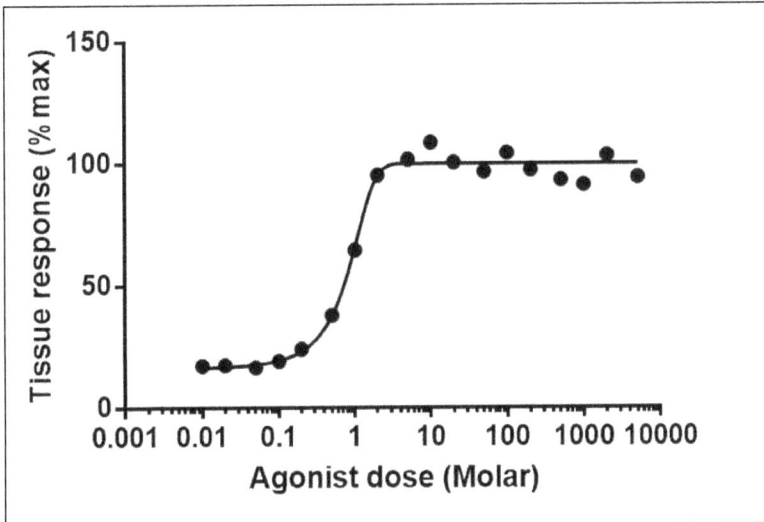

A dose response curve showing the normalised tissue response to stimulation by an agonist. Low doses are insufficient to generate a response, while high doses generate a maximal response. The steepest point of the curve corresponds with an EC50 of 0.7 molar.

Motivation for Studying Dose-response Relationships

Studying dose response, and developing dose–response models, is central to determining safe, hazardous and (where relevant) beneficial levels and dosages for drugs, pollutants, foods, and other substances to which humans or other organisms are exposed. These conclusions are often the basis for public policy. The U.S. Environmental Protection Agency has developed extensive guidance and reports on dose–response modeling and assessment, as well as software. The U.S. Food and Drug Administration also has guidance to elucidate dose–response relationships during drug development. Dose response relationships may be used in individuals or in populations. The adage *The dose makes the poison* reflects how a small amount of a toxin has no significant effect, while a large amount may be fatal. This reflects how dose–response relationships can be used in individuals. In populations, dose–response relationships can describe the way groups of people or organisms are affected at different levels of exposure. Dose response relationships modelled by dose response curves are used extensively in pharmacology and drug development. In particular, the shape of a drug's dose–response curve (quantified by EC50, nH and ymax parameters) reflects the biological activity and strength of the drug.

Example Stimuli and Responses

Some example measures for dose–response relationships are shown in the tables below. Each sensory stimulus corresponds with a particular sensory receptor, for instance the nicotinic acetylcholine receptor for nicotine, or the mechanoreceptor for mechanical pressure. However, stimuli (such as temperatures or radiation) may also affect physiological processes beyond sensation (and even give the measurable response of death). Responses can be recorded as continuous data (e.g. force of muscle contraction) or discrete data (e.g. number of deaths).

Example Stimulus		Target
Drug/Toxin dose	Agonist(e.g. nicotine, isoprenaline)	Biochemical receptors, Enzymes,Transporters
	Antagonist(e.g. ketamine, propranolol)	
	Allosteric modulator (e.g. Benzodiazepine)	
Temperature		Temperature receptors
Sound levels		Hair cells
Illumination/Light intensity		Photoreceptors
Mechanical pressure		Mechanoreceptors
Pathogen dose (e.g. LPS)		n/a
Radiation intensity		n/a

System Level	Example Response
Population (Epidemiology)	Death, loss of consciousness
Organism/Whole animal (Physiology)	Severity of lesion, blood pressure, heart rate, extent of movement, attentiveness, EEG data
Organ/Tissue	ATP production, proliferation, muscle contraction, bile production, cell death
Cell (Cell biology, Biochemistry)	ATP production, calcium signals, morphology, mitosis

Analysis and Creation of Dose-response Curves

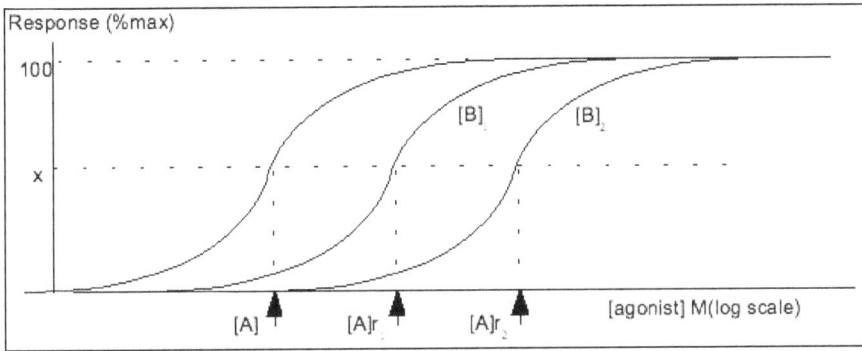

The above figure is a diagrammatic representation of the dose response curves for two concentrations of reversibly competitive antagonist B on the effect of an agonist A. The value taken for response can be any value but typically 50% is used. The first curve is without antagonist, the second two are with increasing concentrations of antagonist.

Semi-log plots of the hypothetical response to agonist, log concentration on the x-axis, in combination with different antagonist concentrations. The parameters of the curves, and how the antagonist changes them, gives useful information about the agonist's pharmacological profile. This curve is similar but distinct from that, which is generated with the ligand-bound receptor concentration on the y-axis.

Construction of Dose-response Curves

A dose–response curve is a coordinate graph relating the magnitude of a stimulus to the response of the receptor. A number of effects (or endpoints) can be studied. The measured dose is generally plotted on the X axis and the response is plotted on the Y axis. In some cases, it is the logarithm of the dose that is plotted on the X axis, and in such cases the curve is typically sigmoidal, with the steepest portion in the middle. Biologically based models using dose are preferred over the use of log (dose) because the latter can visually imply a threshold dose when in fact there is none.

Statistical analysis of dose–response curves may be performed by regression methods such as the probit model or logit model, or other methods such as the Spearman-Karber method. Empirical models based on nonlinear regression are usually preferred over the use of some transformation of the data that linearizes the dose-response relationship.

The organ bath preparation is a typical experimental design for measuring dose-response relationships.

Hill Equation

Dose–response curves are generally sigmoidal and monophasic and can be fit to a classical Hill equation. The Hill equation is a logistic function with respect to the logarithm of the dose and is similar to a logit model. A generalized model for multiphasic cases has also been suggested.

The Hill equation is the following formula, where E is the magnitude of the response, $[A]$ is the drug concentration (or equivalently, stimulus intensity) and EC_{50} is the drug concentration that produces a 50% maximal response and n in the Hill coefficient.

$$\frac{E}{E_{max}} = \frac{1}{1+\left(\dfrac{EC_{50}}{|A|}\right)^{n}}$$

The parameters of the dose response curve reflect measures of potency (such as EC50, IC50, ED50, etc.) and measures of efficacy (such as tissue, cell or population response).

A commonly used dose–response curve is the EC_{50} curve, the half maximal effective concentration, where the EC_{50} point is defined as the inflection point of the curve.

Dose response curves are typically fitted to the Hill equation.

The first point along the graph where a response above zero (or above the control response) is reached is usually referred to as a threshold dose. For most beneficial or recreational drugs, the desired effects are found at doses slightly greater than the threshold dose. At higher doses, undesired side effects appear and grow stronger as the dose increases. The more potent a particular substance is, the steeper this curve will be. In quantitative situations, the Y-axis often is designated by percentages, which refer to the percentage of exposed individuals registering a standard response (which may be death, as in LD_{50}). Such a curve is referred to as a quantal dose–response curve, distinguishing it from a graded dose–response curve, where response is continuous (either measured, or by judgment).

The Hill equation can be used to describe dose–response relationships, for example ion channel-open-probability vs. ligand concentration.

Dose is usually in milligrams, micrograms, or grams per kilogram of body-weight for oral exposures or milligrams per cubic meter of ambient air for inhalation exposures. Other dose units include moles per body-weight, moles per animal, and for dermal exposure, moles per square centimeter.

Limitations

The concept of linear dose–response relationship, thresholds, and all-or-nothing responses may not apply to non-linear situations. A threshold model or linear no-threshold model may be more appropriate, depending on the circumstances. A recent critique of these models as they apply to endocrine disruptors argues for a substantial revision of testing and toxicological models at low doses because of observed non-monotonicity, i.e. U-shaped dose/response curves.

Dose–response relationships generally depend on the exposure time and exposure route (e.g. inhalation, dietary intake); quantifying the response after a different exposure time or for a different route leads to a different relationship and possibly different conclusions on the effects of the stressor under consideration. This limitation is caused by the complexity of biological systems and the often unknown biological processes operating between the external exposure and the adverse cellular or tissue response.

SCHILD REGRESSION

In pharmacology, Schild regression analysis, named for Heinz Otto Schild, is a tool for studying the effects of agonists and antagonists on the response caused by the receptor or on ligand-receptor binding.

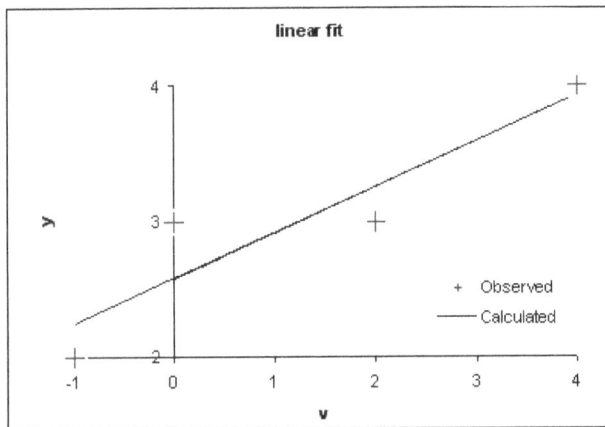

A straight line graph fitted to hypothetical points. The Schild plot of a reversible competitive antagonist should be a straight line, with linear gradient, whose y-intercept relates to the strength of the antagonist.

Dose-response curves can be constructed to describe response or ligand-receptor complex formation as a function of the ligand concentration. Antagonists make it harder to form these complexes by inhibiting interactions of the ligand with its receptor. This is seen as a change in the dose response curve: typically a rightward shift or a lowered maximum. A reversible competitive antagonist should cause a rightward shift in the dose response curve, such that the new curve is parallel to the old one and the maximum is unchanged. This is because reversible competitive antagonists are surmountable antagonists. The magnitude of the rightward shift can be quantified with the dose ratio, r. The dose ratio r is the ratio of the dose of agonist required for half maximal response with the antagonist B present divided by the agonist required for half maximal response without antagonist ("control"). In other words, the ratio of the EC50s of the inhibited and un-inhibited curves. Thus, r represents both the strength of an antagonist and the concentration of the antagonist that was applied. An equation derived from the Gaddum equation can be used to relate r to $[B]$, as follows:

$$r = 1 + \frac{[B]}{K_B}$$

where:

- r is the dose ratio.

- $[B]$ is the concentration of the antagonist.

- K_B is the equilibrium constant of the binding of the antagonist to the receptor.

A Schild plot is a double logarithmic plot, typically $\log_{10}(r-1)$ as the ordinate and $\log_{10}[B]$ as the abscissa. This is done by taking the base-10 logarithm of both sides of the previous equation after subtracting 1:

$$\log_{10}(r-1) = \log_{10}[B] - \log_{10}(K_B)$$

This equation is linear with respect to $\log_{10}[B]$, allowing for easy construction of graphs without computations. This was particular valuable before the use of computers in pharmacology became widespread. The y-intercept of the equation represents the negative logarithm of K_B and can be used to quantify the strength of the antagonist.

These experiments must be carried out on a very wide range (therefore the logarithmic scale) as the mechanisms differ over a large scale, such as at high concentration of drug.

The fitting of the Schild plot to observed data points can be done with regression analysis.

Schild Regression for Ligand Binding

Although most experiments use cellular response as a measure of the effect, the effect is, in essence, a result of the binding kinetics; so, in order to illustrate the mechanism, ligand binding is used. A ligand A will bind to a receptor R according to an equilibrium constant:

$$K_d = \frac{k_{-1}}{k_1}$$

Although the equilibrium constant is more meaningful, texts often mention its inverse, the affinity constant ($K_{aff} = k_1/k_{-1}$): A better binding means an increase of binding affinity.

The equation for simple ligand binding to a single homogeneous receptor is:

$$[AR] = \frac{[R]t[A]}{[A] + K_d}$$

This is the Hill-Langmuir equation, which is practically the Hill equation (biochemistry) described for the agonist binding. In chemistry, this relationship is called the Langmuir equation, which describes the adsorption of molecules onto sites of a surface.

[R]total is the total number of binding sites, and when the equation is plotted it is the horizontal asymptote to which the plot tends; more binding sites will be occupied as the ligand concentration increases, but there will never be 100% occupancy. The binding affinity is the concentration needed to occupy 50% of the sites; the lower this value is the easier it is for the ligand to occupy the binding site.

The binding of the ligand to the receptor at equilibrium follows the same kinetics as an enzyme at steady-state (Michaelis-Menten equation) without the conversion of the bound substrate to product.

Agonists and antagonists can have various effects on ligand binding. They can change the maximum number of binding sites, the affinity of the ligand to the receptor, both effects together or even more bizarre effects when the system being studied is more intact, such as in tissue samples. Tissue absorption, desensitization, and other non equilibrium steady-state can be a problem.

A surmountable drug changes the binding affinity:

- Competitive ligand: $K'_d = K_d \dfrac{1+[B]}{K_b}$

- Cooperative allosteric ligand: $K'_d = K_d \dfrac{K_B+[B]}{K_B+\dfrac{[B]}{\alpha}}$

A nonsurmountable drug changes the maximum binding:

- Noncompetitive binding: $[R]t' = \dfrac{[R]t}{1+\dfrac{[B]}{K_b}}$

- Irreversible binding

The Schild regression also can reveal if there are more than one type of receptor and it can show if the experiment was done wrong as the system has not reached equilibrium.

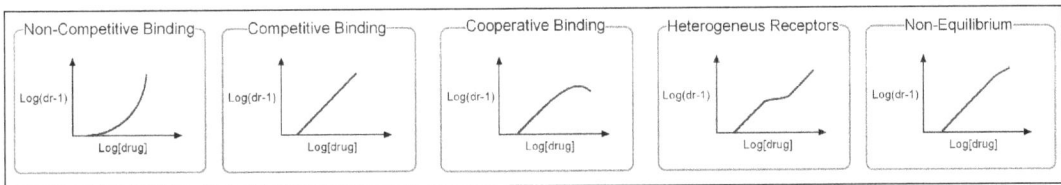

Radioligand Binding Assays

The first radio-receptor assay (RRA) was done in 1970 by Lefkowitz et al. using a radiolabeled hormone to determine the binding affinity for its receptor.

A radio-receptor assay requires the separation of the bound from the free ligand. This is done by filtration, centrifugation or dialysis.

A method that does not require separation is the scintillation proximity assay that relies on the fact that β-rays from ^{3}H travel extremely short distances. The receptors are bound to beads coated with a polyhydroxy scintillator. Only the bound ligands to be detected.

Today, the fluorescence method is preferred to radioactive materials due to a much lower cost, lower hazard, and the possibility of multiplexing the reactions in a high-throughput manner. One problem is that fluorescent-labeled ligands have to bear a bulky fluorophore that may cause it to hinder the ligand binding. Therefore, the fluorophore used, the length of the linker, and its position must be carefully selected.

An example is by using FRET, where the ligand's fluorophore transfers its energy to the fluorophore of an antibody raised against the receptor.

Other detection methods such as surface plasmon resonance do not even require fluorophores.

ANTIMICROBIAL PHARMACODYNAMICS

Antimicrobial pharmacodynamics is the relationship between concentration of antibiotic and its ability to inhibit vital processes of endo- or ectoparasites and microbial organisms. This branch of pharmacodynamics relates concentration of an anti-infective agent to effect, but specifically to its antimicrobial effect.

Concentration-dependent Effects

The minimum inhibitory concentration and minimum bactericidal concentration are used to measure in vitro activity antimicrobial and is an excellent indicator of antimicrobial potency. They don't give any information relating to time-dependent antimicrobial killing the so-called post antibiotic effect.

Post Antibiotic Effect

The post antibiotic effect (PAE) is defined as persistent suppression of bacterial growth after a brief exposure (1 or 2 hours) of bacteria to an antibiotic even in the absence of host defense mechanisms. Factors that affect the duration of the post antibiotic effect include duration of antibiotic exposure, bacterial species, culture medium and class of antibiotic. It has been suggested that an alteration of DNA function is possibly responsible for post antibiotic effect following the observation that most inhibitors of protein and nucleic acid synthesis (aminoglycosides, fluoroquinolones, tetracyclines, clindamycin, certain newer macrolides/ketolides, and rifampicin and rifabutin) induce long-term PAE against susceptible bacteria. Theoretically, the ability of an antibiotic to induce a PAE is an attractive property of an antibiotic since antibiotic concentrations could fall below the MIC for the bacterium yet retain their effectiveness in their ability to suppress the growth. Therefore, an antibiotic with PAE would require less frequent administration and it could improve patient adherence with regard to pharmacotherapy. Proposed mechanisms include slow recovery after reversible nonlethal damage to cell structures; persistence of the drug at a binding site or within the periplasmic space; and the need to synthesize new enzymes before growth can resume. Most antimicrobials possess significant in vitro PAEs ($\geq$ 1.5 hours) against susceptible gram-positive cocci . Antimicrobials with significant PAEs against susceptible gram-negative bacilli are limited to carbapenems and agents that inhibit protein or DNA synthesis.

PHARMACODYNAMIC MODELING

Pharmacodynamic modeling is based on a quantitative integration of pharmacokinetics, pharmacological systems, and (patho-) physiological processes for understanding the intensity and time-course of drug effects on the body. Application of such models to the analysis of meaningful experimental data allows for the quantification and prediction of drug–system interactions for both therapeutic and adverse drug responses.

Useful pharmacodynamic models are based on plausible mathematical and pharmacological exposure–response relationships. Basic model components encompassing a range of pharmacodynamic systems are illustrated in figure. For most drug effects, both pharmacological mechanisms, often characterized by sensitivity-grounded capacity-limited effector units, and physiological turnover processes need to be integrated with drug disposition when constructing a PK/PD model.

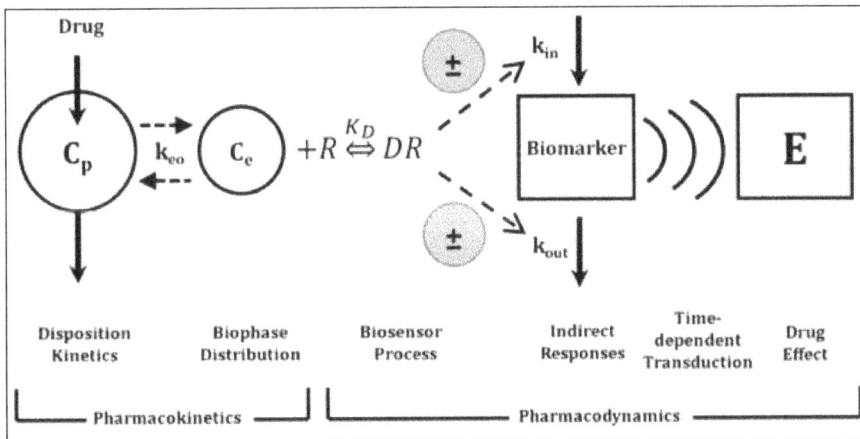

Basic components of pharmacodynamic models. The time-course of drug concentrations in a relevant biological fluid (e.g. plasma, C_p) or the biophase (C_e) is characterized by a mathematical function that serves to drive PD models. The biosensor process involves the interaction between the drug and the pharmacologic target (R), and may be described using various receptor-occupancy models, may require equations that consider the kinetics of the drug–receptor complex formation and dissociation, or may encompass irreversible drug–target interactions. Many drugs act via indirect mechanisms and the biosensor process may serve to stimulate or inhibit the production (k_{in}) or loss (k_{out}) of endogenous mediators. These altered mediators may not represent the final observed drug effect (E) and further time-dependent transduction processes may occur, thus requiring additional modeling components. System complexities such as drug interactions, functional adaptation, changes with pathophysiology, and other factors may play a role in regulating drug effects after acute and long-term drug exposure.

The construction and evaluation of relevant PK/PD models require suitable pharmacokinetic data, an appreciation for molecular and cellular mechanisms of pharmacological/toxicological responses, and a range of quantitative experimental measurements of meaningful biomarkers within the causal pathway between drug–target interactions and clinical effects. Good experimental designs are essential to ensure that sensitive and reproducible data are collected. These data should cover a reasonably wide dose/concentration range and appropriate study duration to ascertain net drug exposure and the ultimate fate of the biomarkers or outcomes under investigation. A wide range of systemic drug concentrations is also typically required for the accurate and precise estimation of pharmacodynamic parameters. Typically studies should involve a minimum of two to three doses to adequately estimate the nonlinear parameters of most pharmacodynamic models with simultaneous collection of concentration and response data. For more complex systems (and therefore models), more extensive datasets are required as these models typically incorporate multiple nonlinear processes and pharmacodynamic endpoints. Models are typically defined using ordinary differential equations and include both drug- and system-specific parameters.

Practical Modeling Approaches

The first steps in any modeling endeavor are to define the objectives of the analysis and to perform a careful graphical analysis of raw data. Both efforts should facilitate selection of appropriate techniques and conditions for model construction and evaluation. A good graphical analysis (along with a priori knowledge of drug mechanisms) may be used to narrow down the number of structural models being considered as a base model and also help in calculating initial parameter estimates. Despite progress in computational algorithms, good initial parameter estimates can reduce the likelihood of falling into local minima and can also be used as a reality check when compared to final parameter estimates or literature reported values. Next, an appropriate drug/toxin pharmacokinetic/toxicokinetic function is derived from fitting a model to concentration–time profiles in relevant biological fluids. Depending on the complexity of the pharmacodynamic model/system, the pharmacokinetic model and associated parameters are often fixed to serve as a driving function for the pharmacodynamic model relating drug exposure to pharmacological/toxicological effects. Although simultaneous PK/PD modeling is desirable, this can still be a formidable challenge for complex models. Objective model-fitting criteria (e.g. diagnostic and goodness-of-fit plots) are frequently compared to select a final model, and a variety of techniques are available to verify or qualify models, which can range in complexity depending on the modeling approach (e.g. population versus pooled data). Ideally, an external dataset, not used in the construction of the model, could be used to determine whether the model is generalizable; however, internal validation steps are far more common as most model-builders will attempt to incorporate all available experimental data. In any event, final models should reasonably recapitulate the data used to derive the model, generate new insights and testable hypotheses of factors controlling drug responses, and provide guidance for subsequent decisions in drug discovery, development, and pharmacotherapy.

Simple Direct Effect Models

The Hill equation assumes that drugs effects (E) are directly proportional to receptor occupancy (i.e. linear transduction), assumes that plasma drug concentrations are in rapid equilibrium with the effect site, and represents a fundamental pharmacodynamic relationship:

$$E = E_0 \pm \frac{E_{max} \times C_p}{EC_{50} + C_p}.$$

This equation, also known as the E_{max} model, describes the concentration–effect relationship in terms of a baseline effect or E_0 (if applicable), the maximum possible effect (E_{max}), and the drug concentration producing half maximal effect (EC_{50}). These parameters can be visualized easily from a plot of effect versus log- concentration where E_{max} is the plateau at relatively high concentrations and EC_{50} is the drug concentration associated with $E = 0.5 \times E_{max}$. Signature temporal profiles for simple direct effects for a compound with monoexponential disposition are shown in figure. The effect versus time curves appear saturated at high dose levels, decline linearly and in parallel over a range of doses, and the peak response time corresponds with the time of peak drug concentrations.

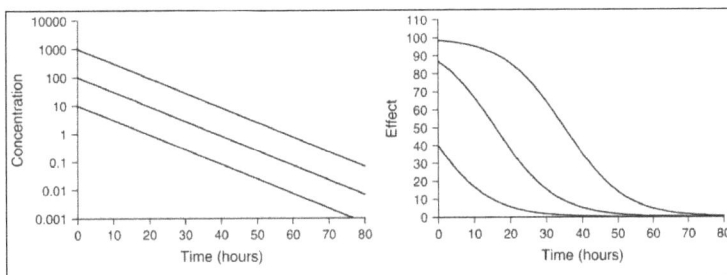

Simulated drug concentrations (left) and response curves (right) using a simple E_{max} model $E = E_0 \pm \dfrac{E_{max} \times C_p}{EC_{50} + C_p}$. Drug concentrations follow monoexponential disposition: $C_p = C^0 e^{(-kt)}$. C^0 was set to 10, 100, or 1,000 units to achieve increasing dose levels. Parameter values were k = 0.12/h, E_{max} = 100 units, and EC_{50} = 15 units.

If a sufficient range of concentrations is not achieved, or cannot be obtained for safety reasons, the Hill equation can be reduced to simpler functions. For concentrations significantly less than the EC_{50}, C_p in the denominator of $E = E_0 \pm \dfrac{E_{max} \times C_p}{EC_{50} + C_p}$ is negligible, and drug effect is directly proportional to plasma drug concentrations:

$$E = E_0 \pm S \times C_p,$$

with S as the slope of the relationship. When the effect is between 20 and 80% maximal, according to $E = E_0 \pm \dfrac{E_{max} \times C_p}{EC_{50} + C_p}$., the effect is directly proportional to the log of drug concentrations:

$$E = E_0 \pm m \log C_p,$$

with m as the slope of the relationship. These reduced functions are only valid within certain ranges of drug concentrations relative to drug potency, and hence cannot be extrapolated to identify the maximal pharmacodynamic effect of a compound.

The full Hill equation, or sigmoid E_{max} model, incorporates a curve-fitting parameter, γ, which describes the steepness of the concentration–effect relationship:

$$E = E_0 \pm \frac{E_{max} \times C_P^{\gamma}}{EC_{50}^{\gamma} + C_P^{\gamma}}.$$

Initial estimates for this parameter can be determined using the linear slope of the effect versus log-concentration plot:

$$m = \frac{E_{max} \times \gamma}{4}.$$

As the Hill coefficient increases from 1 to 5, the concentration–effect relationship becomes less graded, and values of 5 tend to result in quantal or all-or-none types of effects. In contrast, values less than 1 produce very shallow slopes.

Simple direct effect models have been utilized to characterize the adverse effects of a number of drugs. Arrhythmias may occur as a side effect of cardiac and noncardiac therapies, and an increasing number of studies are conducted with QTc intervals as the toxico-dynamic endpoint. QTc prolongation in response to citalopram and tacrolimus has been modeled using a simple E_{max} function. The simple E_{max} model incorporating baseline measurements of the dynamic endpoints was also used to model the cardiovascular toxicity of cocaine administration. The model reasonably described the effects of cocaine on multiple endpoints including heart rate and systolic and diastolic blood pressure. Both the E_{max} and sigmoid E_{max} models were evaluated for describing methemoglobin formation from dapsone metabolites; however, fitting criteria were not evaluated to select the best model.

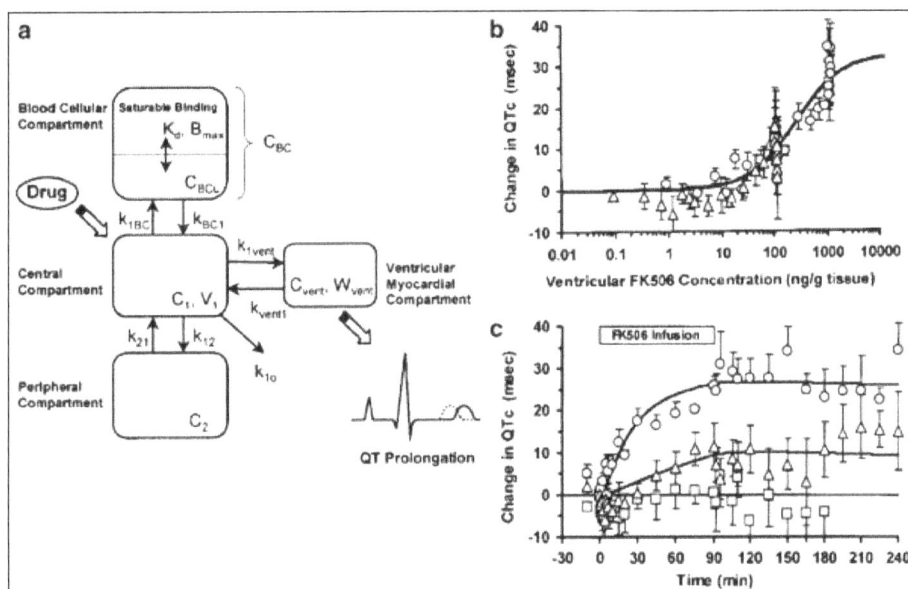

Direct effect model of tacrolimus-induced changes of QTc intervals in guinea pigs. The pharmacokinetic model includes both plasma and ventricular myocardial drug concentrations (a), and the latter are associated with changes in QTc according to

$$E = E_0 \pm \frac{E_{max} \times C_P^{\gamma}}{EC_{50}^{\gamma} + C_P^{\gamma}}.$$ (b). The PK/PD relationship results in the time-course of changes

in QTc (c).

Biophase Distribution

In many cases, the in vivo pharmacological effects will lag behind plasma drug concentrations. This results in the phenomenon of hysteresis, or a temporal disconnect in effect versus concentration plots. Distribution of drug to its site of action might represent a rate-limiting process that may account for the delay in drug effect. The term "biophase" was coined by Furchgott to describe the drug site of action, and a mathematical approach to linking plasma concentrations and drug effect through a hypothetical effect compartment was popularized by Sheiner and colleagues. Plasma drug concentrations are described using an appropriate pharmacokinetic model, and the rate of change of drug concentrations at the biophase (C_e) is defined as:

$$\frac{dC_e}{dt} = k_{eo} \times C_p - k_{eo} \times C_e,$$

with k_{eo} as a first-order distribution rate constant. Although separate rate constants for production and loss were first proposed, they are often set as the same term (k_{eo}) for identifiability purposes. The amount of drug moving into and out of this compartment is assumed to be negligible, and therefore does not influence the pharmacokinetics of the drug. Biophase distribution is combined with $E = E_0 \pm \frac{E_{max} \times C_p}{EC_{50} + C_p}$. or $E = E_0 \pm \frac{E_{max} \times C_P^\gamma}{EC_{50}^\gamma + C_P^\gamma}$., with C_e from $\frac{dC_e}{dt} = k_{eo} \times C_p - k_{eo} \times C_e$, replacing C_p to drive the pharmacological effect.

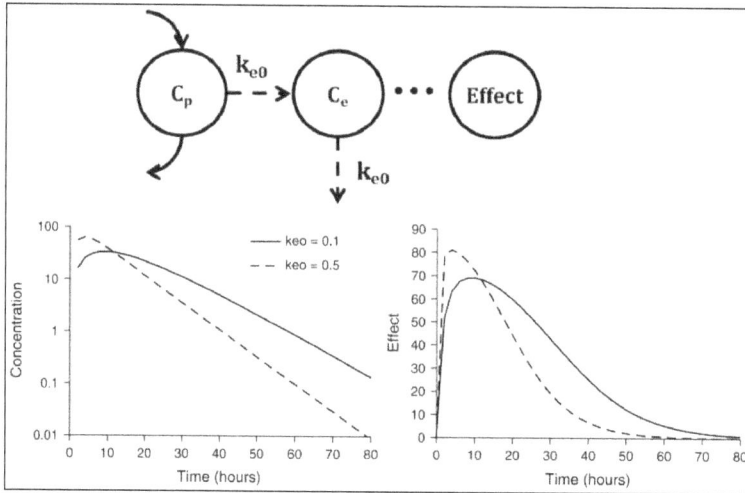

Biophase model structure (top panel) and signature profiles for drug concentrations at the biophase (left bottom panel) and pharmacological effects (right bottom panel). Response curves were simulated using $E = E_0 \pm \frac{E_{max} \times C_p}{EC_{50} + C_p}$. and $\frac{dC_e}{dt} = k_{eo} \times C_p - k_{eo} \times C_e,$ driven by drug concentrations following monoexponential disposition: $C_p = C^o e^{(-kt)}$. C^o was set to 100 units. Parameter values were k = 0.12/h, k_{eo} = 0.1 or 0.5/h, E_{max} = 100 units, and EC_{50} = 15 units.

Figure illustrates the signature profile of the biophase model (i.e. biophase concentration and effect profiles) for a drug exhibiting monoexponential disposition. Peak drug effects are delayed relative to peak plasma concentrations; however, the time to peak effect is observed at the same time, independent of the dose level. The time to peak drug effect is related to k_{eo}, with smaller values resulting in later peak effects. Furthermore, for large dose levels, the slope of the decline of effect is linear and parallel between 20 and 80% of the maximum effect. Estimation of biophase model parameters can be done sequentially by fitting the pharmacokinetics and then fitting the biophase and pharmacodynamic parameters, or by simultaneously fitting all terms.

The biophase model is only suitable for describing delayed responses due to drug distribution. As it was the first approach for describing such delayed drug responses, it has been commonly misapplied to describe systems in which the rate-limiting step is unrelated to drug distribution, resulting in poor fitting and/or unrealistic parameter values.

The biophase model was implemented for describing buprenorphine-induced respiratory depression in rats, and the clinical prediction of transient increases in blood pressure. Yassen and colleagues utilized biophase distribution combined with a sigmoidal E_{max} model to characterize changes in ventilation following a range of dose levels of buprenorphine. In contrast, increases in blood pressure resulting from a drug in clinical development were described using the biophase model coupled with a more complex pharmacodynamic relationship incorporating changes from a blood pressure set point.

Indirect Response Models

Indirect response models represent a highly useful class of models wherein reversible drug–receptor interactions serve to alter the natural production or loss of biomarker response variables. A model reflecting inhibition of production was first utilized to characterize prothrombin activity in blood after oral warfarin administration. Dayneka and colleagues were the first to formally propose four basic indirect response models whose structures are detailed in figure (top panel). These models have been used to investigate the pharmacodynamics of a wide range of drug effects, and their mathematical properties have been well characterized. The four basic models include inhibition of production (Model I) or dissipation (Model II) of response or stimulation of production (Model III) or dissipation of response (Model IV), and are defined by the following differential equations:

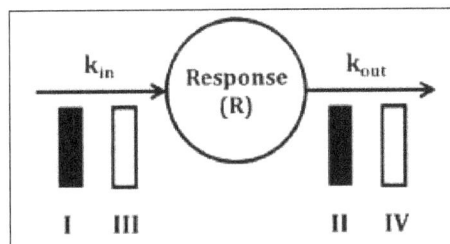

Indirect response model structure (top panel) and signature profiles for the four basic indirect response models (middle and bottom panels). Response curves were simulated using $\quad \dfrac{dR}{dt} = k_{in}\left(1 - \dfrac{I_{max} \times C_p}{IC_{50} + C_p}\right) - k_{out} \times R.,\qquad \dfrac{dR}{dt} = k_{in} - k_{out}\left(1 - \dfrac{I_{max} \times C_p}{IC_{50} + C_p}\right)R.,$

$\dfrac{dR}{dt} = k_{in}\left(1 + \dfrac{S_{max} \times C_p}{SC_{50} + C_p}\right) - k_{out}R.$ and $\dfrac{dR}{dt} = k_{in} - k_{out}\left(1 + \dfrac{S_{max} \times C_p}{SC_{50} + C_p}\right)R,$ driven by drug

concentrations following monoexponential disposition: $C_p = C^o e^{(-kt)}$. C^o was set to 10, 100, or 1,000 units to achieve increasing doses. Parameter values were $k = 0.12/h$, $I_{max} = 1$ unit (Models I and II), $S_{max} = 10$ units (Models III and IV), $EC_{50} = 15$ units, $k_{out} = 0.25/h$, and $R^o = 100$ units ($k_{in} = R^o k_{out}$).

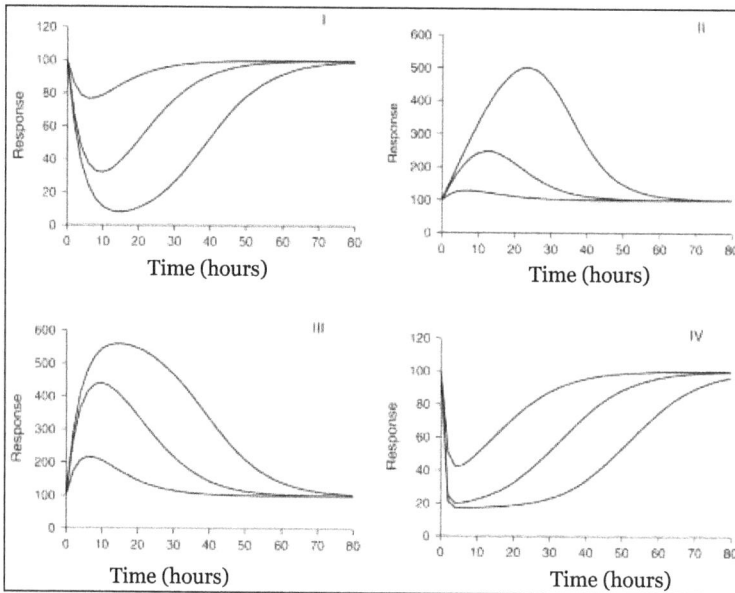

Model I:

$$\frac{dR}{dt} = k_{in}\left(1 - \frac{I_{max} \times C_p}{IC_{50} + C_p}\right) - k_{out} \times R.$$

Model II:

$$\frac{dR}{dt} = k_{in} - k_{out}\left(1 - \frac{I_{max} \times C_p}{IC_{50} + C_p}\right)R.$$

Model III:

$$\frac{dR}{dt} = k_{in}\left(1 + \frac{S_{max} \times C_p}{SC_{50} + C_p}\right) - k_{out}R.$$

Model IV:

$$\frac{dR}{dt} = k_{in} - k_{out}\left(1 + \frac{S_{max} \times C_p}{SC_{50} + C_p}\right)R,$$

where k_{in} is a zero-order production rate constant, k_{out} is a first-order elimination rate constant, I_{max} and S_{max} are defined as the maximum fractional factors of inhibition (o $< I_{max} \le 1$) or stimulation ($S_{max} > 0$), and IC_{50} and SC_{50} are defined as the EC_{50}. Initial parameter estimates can be obtained from a graphical analysis of PK/PD data as previously described. Signature profiles for these models in response to increasing dose levels are shown in figure (middle and bottom panels). Interestingly, the time to peak responses are dose dependent, occurring at later times as the dose level is increased. This phenomenon is easily explained as the inhibition or stimulation effect will continue for larger doses, as drug remains above the EC_{50} for longer times. The initial condition for all models (R_o) is k_{in}/k_{out} which may be set constant or fitted as a parameter during model development. Ideally, a number of measurements should be obtained prior to drug administration to assess baseline conditions. Based on the determinants of R_o, typically the baseline and one of the turnover parameters are estimated, and the remaining rate constant is calculated as a function of the two estimated terms. This reduces the number of parameters to be estimated and maintains system stationarity.

The basic indirect response models can be extended to incorporate a precursor compartment (P). The following equations represent a general set of precursor-dependent indirect response models that were developed and characterized by Sharma and colleagues:

$$\frac{dP}{dt} = K_o\{1 \pm H_1(C_p)\} - (k_s + k_p\{1 \pm H_2(C_p)\})P,$$

$$\frac{dR}{dt} = K_p\{1 \pm H_2(C_p)\} \times P - k_{out} \times R,$$

where k_o represents the zero-order rate constant for precursor production, k_p is a first-order rate constant for production of the response variable, and k_{out} is the first-order rate constant for dissipation of response. H_1 and H_2 represent the inhibition or stimulation of precursor production or production of response and are analogous to the I_{max} and S_{max} functions presented in $\frac{dR}{dt} = k_{in}\left(1 - \frac{I_{max} \times C_p}{IC_{50} + C_p}\right) - k_{out} \times R.$ through $\frac{dR}{dt} = k_{in} - k_{out}\left(1 + \frac{S_{max} \times C_p}{SC_{50} + C_p}\right)R,$. Stimulation or inhibition of k_p is more commonly observed than alterations in the production of precursor. The signature profiles for models V and VI are shown in figure (bottom panels) and clearly demonstrate the rebound effect as drug washes out of the system. The data requirements for these models are similar to the basic indirect response models; however, sufficient data are needed to adequately capture baseline, maximum, and rebound effects, as well as the eventual gradual return to baseline conditions. Responses should be evaluated for two to three doses, with a sufficiently large dose to capture the maximum effect. The response measurements for the large dose should be used to determine initial parameter estimates followed by simultaneous fitting of all response data.

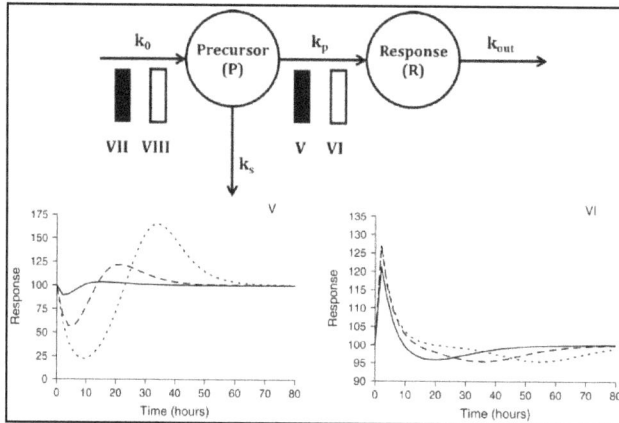

Multiple compartment indirect response models (top panel) and signature profiles for Models V and VI (bottom panel). Response curves were simulated using

$$\frac{dP}{dt} = K_o\{1 \pm H_1(C_p)\} - (k_s + k_p\{1 \pm H_2(C_p)\})P, \text{ and } \frac{dR}{dt} = K_p\{1 \pm H_2(C_p)\} \times P - k_{out} \times R,$$

driven by drug concentrations following monoexponential disposition: $C_p = C^o e^{(-kt)}$. C^o was set to 10, 100, or 1,000 units to achieve increasing doses. Parameter values were k = 0.12/h, I_{max} = 1 unit, S_{max} = 10 units, EC_{50} = 15 units, k_o = 25 unit/h, k_p = 0.5/h, and k_{out} = 0.25/h.

Indirect response models have been utilized to describe the pharmacodynamic effects of a wide range of compounds that alter the natural bioflux or turnover of endogenous substances or functions. A basic indirect response model for erythropoietin was extended to include multiple-compartments for describing the turnover of red blood cells and carboplatin-induced anemia.

This model nicely illustrates the development of a more complex model based on indirect mechanisms of drug action to simultaneously describe multiple in vivo processes.

Signal Transduction Models

Substantial time-delays in the observed pharmacodynamic response may result from multiple time-dependent steps occurring between drug–receptor binding and the ultimate pharmacological response. A transit compartment approach can be utilized to describe a lag between drug concentration and observed effects owing to time-dependent signal transduction. Assuming rapid receptor binding, the following differential equation describes the rate of change of the initial transit compartment (M_1):

$$\frac{dM_1}{dt} = \frac{1}{\tau}\left(\frac{E_{max} \times C_p}{EC_{50} + C_p} - M_1\right),$$

wherein the E_{max} model describes the drug–receptor interaction, and τ is the mean transit time through this compartment. Subsequent transit compartments may be added, and a general equation for the ith compartment can be defined as:

$$\frac{dM_i}{dt} = \frac{1}{\tau}(M_{i-1} - M_i).$$

Later compartments will show a clear delay in the onset of response as well as substantial delays in achieving the maximum effect. Model development for signal transduction systems typically includes evaluating varied numbers of transit compartments and values for τ to determine the combination that best describes the data.

Chemotherapy-induced myelosuppression represents a classic example of the use of a transit compartment modeling to describe this adverse reaction to numerous chemotherapeutic agents . The structural model was proposed by Friberg and colleagues to describe myelosuppression induced by irinotecan, vinflunine , and 2'-deoxy-2'-methylidenecyti-dine for a range of dose levels and various dosing regimens. This same structural model has been used to describe indisulam-induced mye-losuppression, as well as the drug–drug interactions between indisulam and capecitabine, and pemetrexed and BI2536.

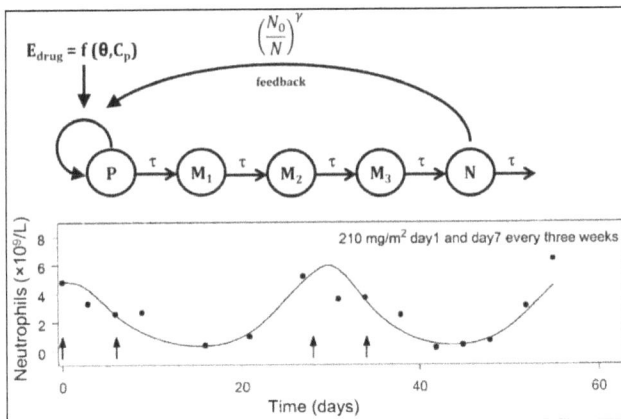

Transit-compartment model of myelosuppression (top panel) including a proliferating progenitor pool (P), three transit compartments (M_i), and a plasma neutrophil compartment (N). Drug effect is driven by plasma drug concentration (C_p) and pharmacodynamic parameters (θ). An adaptive feedback function on the proliferation rate constant is governed by the ratio of initial neutrophils to current neutrophil count, raised to a power coefficient (γ). The time-course of neutrophils following vinflunine administration (arrows in bottom panel).

Irreversible Effect Models

A wide range of compounds, including anticancer drugs, antimicrobial drugs, and enzyme inhibitors, elicit irreversible effects. A basic model for describing irreversible effects was developed by Jusko and includes simple cell killing:

$$\frac{dR}{dt} = -k \times C \times R,$$

where R represents cells or receptors, C is either C_p or C_e, and k is a second-order cell-kill rate constant. The initial condition for this equation is the initial number of cells present within the system (R_0) often represented as a survival fraction. This approach is only applicable for non-proliferating cell populations, but may be extended to incorporate cell growth:

$$\frac{dR}{dt} = k_s \times R - k \times C \times R,$$

with k_s as an apparent first-order growth rate for proliferating cell populations, such as malignant cells or bacteria. This growth rate constant represents the net combination of natural growth and degradation of the cellular population, and its initial estimate can be determined from a control- or nondrug-treated cell population. The model diagram and corresponding signature profiles are shown in figure. The initial slope of the log survival fraction versus time curve out to time, t, and the plasma drug $AUC_{(o-t)}$ can be used to obtain an initial estimate for k ($k = -\ln S_{Ft}/AUC_{(o-t)}$), and the initial condition for equation above is the total cell population at time zero. In contrast to simple cell killing, the effect–time profiles are characterized by an initial cell kill phase, followed by an exponential growth phase, once drug concentrations are below an effective concentration. Clearly the control group is needed to properly characterize the exponential growth rate constant in the untreated cell population.

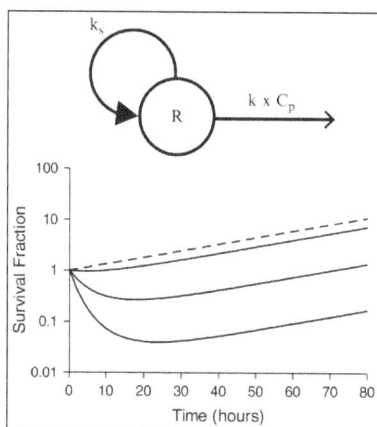

The above figure is a structural model for irreversible effects (top panel) and signature profiles forirreversible effect model with a proliferating cell population (bottom panel).

Response curves were simulated using $\frac{dR}{dt} = k_s \times R - k \times C \times R,$ driven by drug concentrations following monoexponential disposition: $C_p = C^o e^{(-kt)}$. C^o was set to 0, 10, 100, or

1,000 units to achieve a control population and increasing dose levels. Pharmacokinetic parameter was $k = 0.12/h$. Pharmacodynamic parameters were $k = 0.0005$ units/h, $k_s = 0.03/h$.

The irreversible effect model can also be adapted to include the turnover or production and loss of a biomarker:

$$\frac{dR}{dt} = k_{in} - k_{out}R - k \times C \times R.$$

The initial condition for this model is the same as basic indirect responses or k_{in}/k_{out}. The signature profiles for this model are similar to the profiles for indirect response models I and IV It is important to understand the mechanism of action of the response that you are evaluating in order to determine which model should be utilized.

Irreversible effect models are commonly used to describe the cell killing action of chemotherapeutic agents and anti-infectives. This model was also applied to evaluate the formation of methe-moglobin following the administration of a range of antimalarial agents. The final model characterized methemoglobin production resulting from the formation of an active drug metabolite.

More Complex Models

A number of mechanistic processes may be required to adequately describe the drug–system interactions under investigation. Slow receptor binding, tolerance phenomenon, drug interactions, opposing drug effects, and disease progression may add additional complexities to the analysis of toxicodynamic data. For example, Houze and colleagues evaluated paraoxon-induced respiratory toxicity and its reversal with pralidoxime (PRX) administration in rats via the combination of multiple pharmacodynamic modeling components. Initially, the time-course of paraoxon inactivation of in vitro whole blood cholinesterase (WBChE) was modeled based on enzyme inactivation:

$$\frac{dE_A}{dt} = -\left(\frac{kC_{PO}}{EC_{50,PO} + C_{PO}} \right) E_A + k_r E_I,$$

where E_A is active enzyme, k is the maximal rate constant of enzyme inactivation, C_{PO} is paraoxon concentration, $EC_{50,PO}$ is the concentration of paraoxon that produces 50% of k, k_r is a first-order reactivation rate constant, and E_I is the inactive enzyme pool. The rate of change of the inactive enzyme (E_I) was defined as:

$$\frac{dE_I}{dt} = \left(\frac{kC_{PO}}{EC_{50,PO} + C_{PO}}\right)E_A - (k_r + k_{age})E_I,$$

where k_{age} is a first-order rate constant of aging of inactive enzyme. The reactivation of this in vitro system by PRX was modeled as an indirect response, and

$$\frac{dE_A}{dt} = -\left(\frac{kC_{PO}}{EC_{50,PO} + C_{PO}}\right)E_A + k_r E_I, \quad \text{and} \quad \frac{dE_I}{dt} = \left(\frac{kC_{PO}}{EC_{50,PO} + C_{PO}}\right)E_A - (k_r + k_{age})E_I,$$

were updated accordingly:

$$\frac{dE_A}{dt} = \left(\frac{kC_{PO}}{EC_{50,PO} + C_{PO}}\right)E_A + k_r\left(1 + \frac{E_{max}C_{PRX}^h}{EC_{50,PRX}^h + C_{PRX}^h}\right)E_I,$$

$$\frac{dE_I}{dt} = \left(\frac{kC_{PO}}{EC_{50,PO} + C_{PO}}\right)E_A - k_r\left(1 + \frac{E_{max}C_{PRX}^h}{EC_{50,PRX}^h + C_{PRX}^h}\right)E_I$$

Interestingly, the estimated potency of PRX was in agreement with an empirical literature estimate. For the in vivo dynamics, a fixed pharmacokinetic function for PRX was introduced, and an empirical function was used to describe paraoxon-induced enzyme inactivation, as plasma concentrations were unavailable. The estimated parameters from the in vitro analysis were fixed (not identi-fiable from in vivo data only), and the toxicodynamic biomarker, expiratory time (T_E), was linked to apparent active enzyme (E_A) according to the following nonlinear transfer function:

$$T_E = T_E^0 + \frac{E_{max,T_E}\left(\frac{E_0}{E_A} - 1\right)^n}{E_{50}^n + \left(\frac{E_0}{E_A} - 1\right)^n},$$

where T_E^0 is the baseline expiratory time, $E_{max,\ TE}$ is the maximal increase in T_E, E_0 is the baseline active enzyme (1 or 100%), E_{50} is the corrected enzyme ratio resulting in 50% of $E_{max,\ TE}$, and n is a sigmoidicity coefficient.

An additional theoretical example of mechanism-based analysis of drug interactions was presented by Earp and colleagues, who examined drug interactions utilizing indirect response models. These more complex models typically consider multiple pharmaco-dynamic endpoints which require individual data sets and stepwise analysis for each endpoint. A corticosteroid model which considers mRNA dynamics of the glucocorticoid receptor and hepatic tyro-sine aminotransferase mRNA and activity is an example of simultaneously characterizing multiple pharmacodynamic endpoints using an integration of basic modeling components .

The majority of mechanism-based pharmacodynamic models describe continuous physiological response variables. However, models are available for evaluating non-continuous outcomes, such as the probability of a specific event occurring. Such responses are often more clinically relevant, and more research is needed to combine continuous mechanistic PK/PD models with clinical outcomes data. One example is the prediction of enoxaparin-induced bleeding events in patients undergoing various therapeutic dosing regimens . A population proportional-odds model was developed to predict the severity of bleeding event on an ordinal scale of 1–3 .

References

- Ashauer R, Escher B. 2010. Advantages of Toxicokinetic and Toxicodynamic modeling in aquatic ecotoxicology and risk assessment. Journal of Environmental Monitoring 12: 2056-2061

- Drug-action-and-pharmacodynamics, pharmacology-introduction, pharmacology: merckvetmanual.com, Retrieved 27 May, 2019

- Zarrini G, Bahari-Delgosha Z, Mollazadeh-Moghaddam K, Shahverdi AR (2010). "Post-antibacterial effect of thymol". Pharmaceutical Biology. 48 (6): 633–636. Doi:10.3109/13880200903229098. PMID 20645735

- Choi, S.M., Yoo, S.D., Lee, B.M. 2010. Toxicological Characteristics of Endocrine-Disrupting Chemicals: Developmental Toxicity, Carcinogenicity, and Mutagenicity. Journal of Toxicology and Environmental Health, Part B: Critical Reviews, 7:1, 1-23

- C.H. Nightingale, T. Murakawa, P.G. Ambrose (2002) Antimicrobial Pharmacodynamics in Theory and Clinical Practice Informa Health Care ISBN 0-8247-0561-0

5

Psychopharmacology

The scientific study of the effects of drugs on sensation, mood, thinking and behavior is known as psychopharmacology. Some of the psychoactive drugs which are studied within this field are psychiatric medication, benzodiazepine and hallucinogens. All these diverse drugs as well as the role of psychopharmacology in mental health have been carefully analyzed in this chapter.

Psychopharmacology is a field, which analyses the impact of different drugs on the mental health of patients. It considers how different compounds alter people's behavior by changing the way that the person thinks or feels. Some of the conditions that these medicines are used to treat include depression, psychosis and anxiety.

A psychopharmacologist is an expert advisor on which drug might have the best impact on a patient with a particular mental health condition. They understand how the medicine works and what the expected clinical outcomes are. The medic is also likely to have a grasp of neuroscience as the medicines used have impacts on the functioning of the central nervous system. Moreover, they comprehend the differences between a wide range of mental health conditions.

In order to prescribe drugs, the psychopharmacologist will need to have an in depth understanding of the drug's pharmacokinetics (i.e. the movement of the drug within the body) and pharmacodynamics (i.e. the effects of the drug and its mechanism of action). This is particularly important should a medicine interact with any reward regions of the body as the psychopharmacologist would not, for example, want a medicine to interact too quickly and cause the patient to become addicted to a possible high that the medicine gives them.

Therefore, the scientist needs to understand how the drug interacts with the body over time at a particular dose, how long it stays in the body and also if it is likely to react with any other medicines that the patient is taking. They should also have some knowledge of the genetics of patients as well as this may have a significant impact as well.

Neurotransmitters for Psychopharmacology

The drugs used in psychopharmacology have an impact on the neurotransmitters in the brain.

Developments have focused primarily on agents that affect the neurotransmitters for depression, psychoses and anxiety. However, there have been no further major breakthroughs regarding neurotransmitters in recent years.

The key neurotransmitters affected in psychotropic medicines are:

- Acetylcholine involved in the body's learning, memory, mood and also Alzheimer's Disease.

- Dopamine involved in motor circuits for Parkinson's Disease, reward and pleasure centers and Schizophrenia.

- Endogenous opioids such as endorphins and enkephalins involved in pain, analgesia and reward.

- GABA involved in anxiety, epilepsy, fear, stress and inhibitory neurotransmitter diseases.

- Glutamate involved in learning, memory, communication and excitatory neurotransmitter diseases.

- Norepinephrine involved in depression and arousal.

- Serotonin involved in aggression, depression, desire and schizophrenia.

The different types of drugs in mental health management:

Scientific awareness of the type of impact that medicines have on the mental health of people progressed considerably in the 1950s. This was when psychotropic drugs, medicines that alter the way a patient behaves, were discovered. Over the years, a wide range of antidepressants, antianxiety, antimanic, antipsychotics and stimulant drugs have been developed.

- Selective serotonin reuptake inhibitors (SSRIs): Increase serotonin and are often used as antidepressants.

- Antimanic drugs (mood stabilizers): Reduce nerve impulses to manage manic episodes.

- Antianxiety drugs (tranquilizers): Have a calming effect and slow down the central nervous system.

- Serotonin and noradrenaline reuptake inhibitors: These increase the serotonin and noradrenalin.

How Drugs affect Mental Health?

Neurons are cells in the nervous system. There are about 100 billion of them. They communicate information in a chemical (neurotransmitter) and electrical way throughout the body. There are different types of neurons. Sensory neurons send information from sensory receptor cells to the brain. Motor neurons are essential in transmitting information from the brain to the muscles. Also interneurons communicate between neurons.

Neurotransmitters bind to proteins on the receiving neuron and then further communication is possible. The medicines that are used in altering the mental health of patients operate by changing the way that these neurons communicate with one another.

Psychotropic drugs also tend to be amphiphilic molecules meaning that they are soluble in both water and lipids. This helps to ease their interactions in the body.

PSYCHOACTIVE DRUGS

A psychoactive drug, psychopharmaceutical, or psychotropic drug is a chemical substance that changes brain function and results in alterations in perception, mood, consciousness, cognition, or behavior. These substances may be used medically; recreationally; to purposefully improve performance or alter one's consciousness; as entheogens; for ritual, spiritual, or shamanic purposes; or for research. Some categories of psychoactive drugs, which have therapeutic value, are prescribed by physicians and other healthcare practitioners. Examples include anesthetics, analgesics, anticonvulsant and antiparkinsonian drugs as well as medications used to treat neuropsychiatric disorders, such as antidepressants, anxiolytics, antipsychotics, and stimulant medications. Some psychoactive substances may be used in the detoxification and rehabilitation programs for persons dependent on or addicted to other psychoactive drugs.

Psychoactive substances often bring about subjective (although these may be objectively observed) changes in consciousness and mood that the user may find rewarding and pleasant (e.g. euphoria or a sense of relaxation) or advantageous (e.g. increased alertness) and are thus reinforcing. Substances which are both rewarding and positively reinforcing have the potential to induce a state of addiction – compulsive drug use despite negative consequences. In addition, sustained use of some substances may produce physical or psychological dependence or both, associated with somatic or psychological-emotional withdrawal states respectively. Drug rehabilitation attempts to reduce addiction, through a combination of psychotherapy, support groups, and other psychoactive substances. Conversely, certain psychoactive drugs may be so unpleasant that the person will never use the substance again. This is especially true of certain deliriants (e.g. Jimson weed), powerful dissociatives (e.g. *Salvia divinorum*), and classic psychedelics (e.g. LSD, psilocybin), in the form of a "bad trip".

Psychoactive drug misuse, dependence and addiction have resulted in legal measures and moral debate. Governmental controls on manufacture, supply and prescription attempt to reduce problematic medical drug use. Ethical concerns have also been raised about over-use of these drugs clinically, and about their marketing by manufacturers. Popular campaigns to decriminalize or legalize certain recreational drug use (e.g. cannabis) are also ongoing.

Purposes

Psychoactive substances are used by humans for a number of different purposes to achieve a specific end. These uses vary widely between cultures. Some substances may have controlled or illegal uses while others may have shamanic purposes, and still others are used medicinally. Other examples would be social drinking, nootropic, or sleep aids. Caffeine is the world's most widely consumed psychoactive substance, but unlike many others, it is legal and unregulated in nearly all jurisdictions. In North America, 90% of adults consume caffeine daily.

Psychoactive drugs are divided into different groups according to their pharmacological effects. Commonly used psychoactive drugs and groups:

- Anxiolytics.

  Example: Benzodiazepines, barbiturates.

- Empathogen–entactogens.

  Example: MDMA (Ecstasy), MDA, 6-APB, AMT.

- Stimulants ("uppers"). This category comprises substances that wake one up, stimulate the mind, and may cause euphoria, but do not affect perception.

  Examples: Amphetamine, caffeine, cocaine, nicotine, modafinil.

- Depressants ("downers"), including sedatives, hypnotics, and opioids. This category includes all of the calmative, sleep-inducing, anxiety-reducing, anesthetizing substances, which sometimes induce perceptual changes, such as dream images, and also often evoke feelings of euphoria.

  Examples: Ethanol (alcoholic beverages), opioids, cannabis, barbiturates, benzodiazepines.

- Hallucinogens, including psychedelics, dissociatives and deliriants. This category encompasses all those substances that produce distinct alterations in perception, sensation of space and time, and emotional states.

  Examples: Psilocybin, LSD, *Salvia divinorum*, nitrous oxide and scopolamine.

Uses

Anesthesia

General anesthetics are a class of psychoactive drug used on people to block physical pain and other sensations. Most anesthetics induce unconsciousness, allowing the person to undergo medical procedures like surgery without the feelings of physical pain or emotional trauma. To induce unconsciousness, anesthetics affect the GABA and NMDA systems. For example, propofol is a GABA agonist, and ketamine is an NMDA receptor antagonist.

Pain Management

Psychoactive drugs are often prescribed to manage pain. The subjective experience of pain is primarily regulated by endogenous opioid peptides. Thus, pain can often be managed using psychoactives that operate on this neurotransmitter system, also known as opioid receptor agonists. This class of drugs can be highly addictive, and includes opiate narcotics, like morphine and codeine. NSAIDs, such as aspirin and ibuprofen, are also analgesics. These agents also reduce eicosanoid-mediated inflammation by inhibiting the enzyme cyclooxygenase.

Mental Disorders

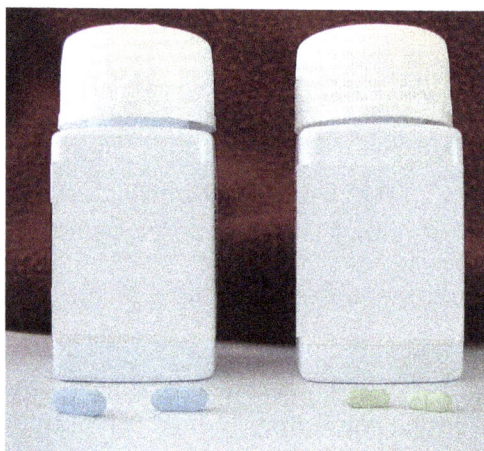

Antidepressant

Psychiatric medications are psychoactive drugs prescribed for the management of mental and emotional disorders, or to aid in overcoming challenging behavior. There are six major classes of psychiatric medications:

- Antidepressants treat disorders such as clinical depression, dysthymia, anxiety, eating disorders and borderline personality disorder.

- Stimulants, used to treat disorders such as attention deficit hyperactivity disorder and narcolepsy, and for weight reduction.

- Antipsychotics, used to treat psychotic symptoms, such as those associated with schizophrenia or severe mania, or as adjuncts to relieve clinical depression.

- Mood stabilizers, used to treat bipolar disorder and schizoaffective disorder.

- Anxiolytics, used to treat anxiety disorders.

- Depressants, used as hypnotics, sedatives, and anesthetics, depending upon dosage.

In addition, several psychoactive substances are currently employed to treat various addictions. These include acamprosate or naltrexone in the treatment of alcoholism, or methadone or buprenorphine maintenance therapy in the case of opioid addiction.

Exposure to psychoactive drugs can cause changes to the brain that counteract or augment some of their effects; these changes may be beneficial or harmful. However, there is a significant amount of evidence that relapse rate of mental disorders negatively corresponds with length of properly followed treatment regimens (that is, relapse rate substantially declines over time), and to a much greater degree than placebo.

Recreation

Many psychoactive substances are used for their mood and perception altering effects, including those with accepted uses in medicine and psychiatry. Examples of psychoactive substances include caffeine, alcohol, cocaine, LSD, nicotine and cannabis. Classes of drugs frequently used recreationally include:

- Stimulants, which activate the central nervous system. These are used recreationally for their euphoric effects.

- Hallucinogens (psychedelics, dissociatives and deliriants), which induce perceptual and cognitive alterations.

- Hypnotics, which depress the central nervous system.

- Opioid analgesics, which also depress the central nervous system. These are used recreationally because of their euphoric effects.

- Inhalants, in the forms of gas aerosols, or solvents, which are inhaled as a vapor because of their stupefying effects. Many inhalants also fall into the above categories (such as nitrous oxide which is also an analgesic).

In some modern and ancient cultures, drug usage is seen as a status symbol. Recreational drugs are seen as status symbols in settings such as at nightclubs and parties. For example, in ancient Egypt, gods were commonly pictured holding hallucinogenic plants.

Because there is controversy about regulation of recreational drugs, there is an ongoing debate about drug prohibition. Critics of prohibition believe that regulation of recreational drug use is a violation of personal autonomy and freedom. In the United States, critics have noted that prohibition or regulation of recreational and spiritual drug use might be unconstitutional, and causing more harm than is prevented.

Ritual and Spiritual

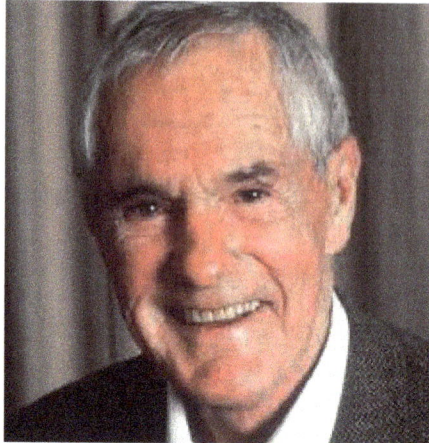

Timothy Leary was a leading proponent of spiritual hallucinogen use.

Certain psychoactives, particularly hallucinogens, have been used for religious purposes since prehistoric times. Native Americans have used peyote cacti containing mescaline for religious ceremonies for as long as 5700 years. The muscimol-containing Amanita muscaria mushroom was used for ritual purposes throughout prehistoric Europe.

The use of entheogens for religious purposes resurfaced in the West during the counterculture movements of the 1960s and 70s. Under the leadership of Timothy Leary, new spiritual and intention-based movements began to use LSD and other hallucinogens as tools to access deeper inner exploration. In the United States, the use of peyote for ritual purposes is protected only for members of the Native American Church, which is allowed to cultivate and distribute peyote. However, the genuine religious use of peyote, regardless of one's personal ancestry, is protected in Colorado, Arizona, New Mexico, Nevada, and Oregon.

Military

Psychoactive drugs have been used in military applications as non-lethal weapons.

Both military and civilian American intelligence officials are known to have used psychoactive drugs while interrogating captives apprehended in its War on Terror. In July 2012, Jason Leopold and Jeffrey Kaye, psychologists and human rights workers, had a Freedom of Information Act request fulfilled that confirmed that the use of psychoactive drugs during interrogation was a long-standing practice. Captives and former captives had been reporting medical staff collaborating with interrogators to drug captives with powerful psychoactive drugs prior to interrogation since the very first captives' release. In May 2003, recently released Pakistani captive Sha Mohammed Alikhel described the routine use of psychoactive drugs in the Guantanamo Bay detention center. He said that Jihan Wali, a captive kept in a nearby cell, was rendered catatonic through the use of these drugs.

The military justice system has also been known to use psychoactive drugs to obtain a conviction.

Additionally, militaries worldwide have used or are using various psychoactive drugs to improve performance of soldiers by suppressing hunger, increasing the ability to sustain effort without food, increasing and lengthening wakefulness and concentration, suppressing fear, reducing empathy, and improving reflexes and memory-recall among other things.

Route of Administration

Psychoactive drugs are administered via oral ingestion as a tablet, capsule, powder, liquid, and beverage; via injection by subcutaneous, intramuscular, and intravenous route; via rectum by suppository and enema; and via inhalation by smoking, vaporization and insufflation ("snorting"). The efficiency of each method of administration varies from drug to drug.

The psychiatric drugs fluoxetine, quetiapine, and lorazepam are ingested orally in tablet or capsule form. Alcohol and caffeine are ingested in beverage form; nicotine and cannabis are smoked or vaped; peyote and psilocybin mushrooms are ingested in botanical form or dried; and crystalline drugs such as cocaine and methamphetamine are usually insufflated (inhaled or "snorted").

Determinants of Effects

The theory of dosage, set, and setting is a useful model in dealing with the effects of psychoactive substances, especially in a controlled therapeutic setting as well as in recreational use. Dr. Timothy Leary, based on his own experiences and systematic observations on psychedelics, developed this theory along with his colleagues Ralph Metzner, and Richard Alpert (Ram Dass) in the 1960s.

Dosage

The first factor, dosage, has been a truism since ancient times, or at least since Paracelsus who said, "Dose makes the poison." Some compounds are beneficial or pleasurable when consumed in small amounts, but harmful, deadly, or evoke discomfort in higher doses.

Set

The set is the internal attitudes and constitution of the person, including their expectations, wishes, fears, and sensitivity to the drug. This factor is especially important for the hallucinogens, which have the ability to make conscious experiences out of the unconscious. In traditional cultures, set is shaped primarily by the worldview, health and genetic characteristics that all the members of the culture share.

Setting

The third aspect is setting, which pertains to the surroundings, the place, and the time in which the experiences transpire.

This theory clearly states that the effects are equally the result of chemical, pharmacological, psychological, and physical influences. The model that Timothy Leary proposed applied to the psychedelics, although it also applies to other psychoactives.

Effects

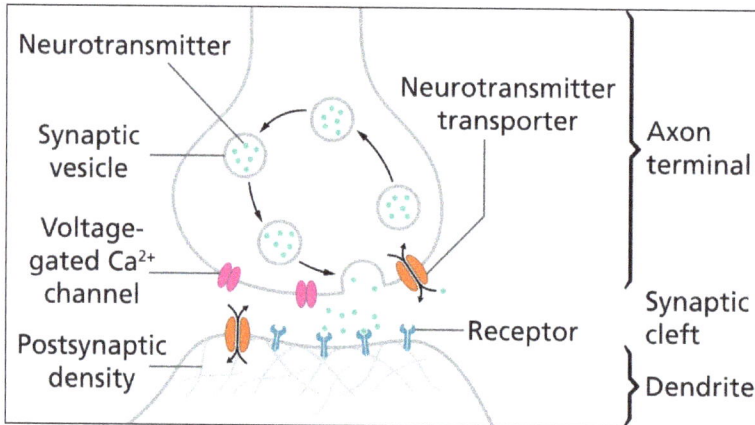

The major elements of neurotransmission. Depending on its method of action, a psychoactive substance may block the receptors on the post-synaptic neuron (dendrite), or block reuptake or affect neurotransmitter synthesis in the pre-synaptic neuron (axon).

Psychoactive drugs operate by temporarily affecting a person's neurochemistry, which in turn causes changes in a person's mood, cognition, perception and behavior. There are many ways in which psychoactive drugs can affect the brain. Each drug has a specific action on one or more neurotransmitter or neuroreceptor in the brain.

Drugs that increase activity in particular neurotransmitter systems are called agonists. They act by increasing the synthesis of one or more neurotransmitters, by reducing its reuptake from the synapses, or by mimicking the action by binding directly to the postsynaptic receptor. Drugs that reduce neurotransmitter activity are called antagonists, and operate by interfering with synthesis or blocking postsynaptic receptors so that neurotransmitters cannot bind to them.

Exposure to a psychoactive substance can cause changes in the structure and functioning of neurons, as the nervous system tries to re-establish the homeostasis disrupted by the presence of the drug. Exposure to antagonists for a particular neurotransmitter can increase the number of receptors for that neurotransmitter or the receptors themselves may become more responsive to neurotransmitters; this is called sensitization. Conversely, overstimulation of receptors for a particular neurotransmitter may cause a decrease in both number and sensitivity of these receptors, a process called desensitization or tolerance. Sensitization and desensitization are more likely to occur with long-term exposure, although they may occur after only a single exposure. These processes are thought to play a role in drug dependence and addiction. Physical dependence on antidepressants or anxiolytics may result in worse depression or anxiety, respectively, as withdrawal symptoms. Unfortunately, because clinical depression (also called major depressive disorder) is often referred to simply as depression, antidepressants are often requested by and prescribed for patients who are depressed, but not clinically depressed.

Addiction and Dependence

Comparison of the perceived harm for various psychoactive drugs from a poll among medical psychiatrists specialized in addiction treatment.

Psychoactive drugs are often associated with addiction or drug dependence. Dependence can be divided into two types: psychological dependence, by which a user experiences negative psychological or emotional withdrawal symptoms (e.g. depression) and physical dependence, by which a user must use a drug to avoid physically uncomfortable or even medically harmful physical withdrawal symptoms. Drugs that are both rewarding and reinforcing are addictive; these properties of a drug are mediated through activation of the mesolimbic dopamine pathway, particularly the nucleus accumbens. Not all addictive drugs are associated with physical dependence, e.g. amphetamine, and not all drugs that produce physical dependence are addictive drugs, e.g. caffeine.

Many professionals, self-help groups, and businesses specialize in drug rehabilitation, with varying degrees of success, and many parents attempt to influence the actions and choices of their children regarding psychoactives.

Common forms of rehabilitation include psychotherapy, support groups and pharmacotherapy, which uses psychoactive substances to reduce cravings and physiological withdrawal symptoms while a user is going through detox. Methadone, itself an opioid and a psychoactive substance, is a common treatment for heroin addiction, as is another opioid, buprenorphine. Recent research on addiction has shown some promise in using psychedelics such as ibogaine to treat and even cure drug addictions, although this has yet to become a widely accepted practice.

Psychiatric Medication

A psychiatric medication is a licensed psychoactive drug taken to exert an effect on the chemical makeup of the brain and nervous system. Thus, these medications are used to treat mental illnesses. Usually prescribed in psychiatric settings, these medications are typically made of synthetic chemical compounds. Since the mid-20th century, such medications have been leading treatments for a broad range of mental disorders and have decreased the need for long-term hospitalization, therefore lowering the cost of mental health care. The recidivism or rehospitalization of the mentally ill is at a high rate in many countries and the reasons for the relapses are under research.

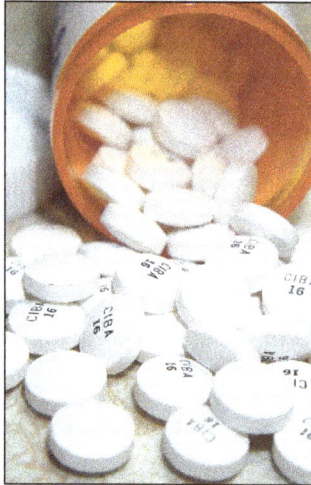

Ritalin sustained-release (SR) 20 mg tablets.

Administration

Psychiatric medications are prescription medications, requiring a prescription from a physician, such as a psychiatrist, or a psychiatric nurse practitioner, PMHNP, before they can be obtained. Some U.S. states and territories, following the creation of the prescriptive authority for psychologists movement, have granted prescriptive privileges to clinical psychologists who have undergone additional specialised education and training in medical psychology. In addition to the familiar dosage in pill form, psychiatric medications are evolving into more novel methods of drug delivery. New technologies include transdermal, transmucosal, inhalation, and suppository supplements.

Psychopharmacology studies a wide range of substances with various types of psychoactive properties. The professional and commercial fields of pharmacology and psychopharmacology do not typically focus on psychedelic or recreational drugs, and so the majority of studies are conducted on psychiatric medication. While studies are conducted on all psychoactive drugs by both fields, psychopharmacology focuses on psychoactive and chemical interactions within the brain. Physicians who research psychiatric medications are psychopharmacologists, specialists in the field of psychopharmacology.

Adverse and Withdrawal Effects

Psychiatric medications carry risk for adverse effects. The occurrence of adverse effects can potentially reduce drug compliance. Some adverse effects can be treated symptomatically by using adjunct medications such as anticholinergics (antimuscarinics). Some rebound or withdrawal adverse effects, such as the possibility of a sudden or severe emergence or re-emergence of psychosis in antipsychotic withdrawal, may appear when the drugs are discontinued, or discontinued too rapidly.

Medicine Combinations with Clinically Untried Risks

While clinical trials of psychiatric medications, like other medications, typically test medicines separately, there is a practice in psychiatry (more so than in somatic medicine) to use polypharmacy in combinations of medicines that have never been tested together in clinical trials (though all medicines involved have passed clinical trials separately). It is argued that this presents a risk of adverse effects, especially brain damage, in real-life mixed medication psychiatry that are not visible in the clinical trials of one medicine at a time (similar to mixed drug abuse causing significantly more damage than the additive effects of brain damages caused by using only one illegal drug). Outside clinical trials, there is evidence for an increase in mortality when psychiatric patients are transferred to polypharmacy with an increased number of medications being mixed.

Types

There are six main groups of psychiatric medications.

- Antidepressants, which treat disparate disorders such as clinical depression, dysthymia, anxiety disorders, eating disorders and borderline personality disorder.

- Antipsychotics, which treat psychotic disorders such as schizophrenia and psychotic symptoms occurring in the context of other disorders such as mood disorders.

- Anxiolytics, which treat anxiety disorders.

- Depressants, which are used as hypnotics, sedatives, and anesthetics.

- Mood stabilizers, which treat bipolar disorder and schizoaffective disorder.

- Stimulants, which treat disorders such as attention deficit hyperactivity disorder and narcolepsy.

Antidepressants

Antidepressants are drugs used to treat clinical depression, and they are also often used for anxiety and other disorders. Most antidepressants will hinder the breakdown of serotonin or norepinephrine or both. A commonly used class of antidepressants are called selective serotonin reuptake inhibitors (SSRIs), which act on serotonin transporters in the brain to increase levels of serotonin in the synaptic cleft. SSRIs will often take 3–5 weeks to have a noticeable effect, as the regulation of receptors in the brain adapts. There are multiple classes of antidepressants which have different mechanisms of action. Another type of antidepressant is a monoamine oxidase inhibitor, which is thought to block the action of Monoamine oxidase, an enzyme that breaks down serotonin and norepinephrine. MAOIs are not used as first-line treatment due to the risk of hypertensive crisis related to the consumption of foods containing the amino acid tyramine.

Common antidepressants:

- Fluoxetine (Prozac), SSRI.

- Paroxetine (Paxil, Seroxat), SSRI.

- Citalopram (Celexa), SSRI.

- Escitalopram (Lexapro), SSRI.

- Sertraline (Zoloft), SSRI.

- Duloxetine (Cymbalta), SNRI.

- Venlafaxine (Effexor), SNRI.

- Bupropion (Wellbutrin), NDRI.

- Mirtazapine (Remeron), NaSSA.

- Isocarboxazid (Marplan), MAOI.

- Phenelzine (Nardil), MAOI.

- Tranylcypromine (Parnate), MAOI.

- Amitriptyline (Elavil), TCA.

Antipsychotics

Antipsychotics are drugs used to treat various symptoms of psychosis, such as those caused by psychotic disorders or schizophrenia. Atypical antipsychotics are also used as mood stabilizers in the treatment of bipolar disorder, and they can augment the action of antidepressants in major depressive disorder. Antipsychotics are sometimes referred to as neuroleptic drugs and some antipsychotics are branded major tranquilizers.

There are two categories of antipsychotics: typical antipsychotics and atypical antipsychotics. Most antipsychotics are available only by prescription.

Common antipsychotics:

Typical antipsychotics	Atypical antipsychotics
• Chlorpromazine (Thorazine)	• Aripiprazole (Abilify)
• Haloperidol (Haldol)	• Clozapine (Clozaril)
• Perphenazine (Trilafon)	• Lurasidone (Latuda)
• Thioridazine (Melleril)	• Olanzapine (Zyprexa)
• Thiothixene (Navane)	• Paliperidone (Invega)
• Flupenthixol (Fluanxol)	• Quetiapine (Seroquel)
• Trifluoperazine (Stelazine)	• Risperidone (Risperdal)
	• Zotepine (Nipolept)
	• Ziprasidone (Geodon)

Anxiolytics and Hypnotics

Benzodiazepines are effective as hypnotics, anxiolytics, anticonvulsants, myorelaxants and amnesics. Having less proclivity for overdose and toxicity, they have widely supplanted barbiturates.

Developed in the 1950s onward, benzodiazepines were originally thought to be non-addictive at therapeutic doses, but are now known to cause withdrawal symptoms similar to barbiturates and alcohol. Benzodiazepines are generally recommended for short-term use.

Z-drugs are a group of drugs with effects generally similar to benzodiazepines, which are used in the treatment of insomnia.

Common benzodiazepines and z-drugs include:

Benzodiazepines	Z-drug hypnotics
• Alprazolam (Xanax), anxiolytic	• Eszopiclone (Lunesta)
• Chlordiazepoxide (Librium), anxiolytic	• Zaleplon (Sonata)
• Clonazepam (Klonopin), anxiolytic	• Zolpidem (Ambien, Stilnox)
• Diazepam (Valium), anxiolytic	• Zopiclone (Imovan)
• Lorazepam (Ativan), anxiolytic	
• Nitrazepam (Mogadon), hypnotic	
• Temazepam (Restoril), hypnotic	

Mood Stabilizers

In 1949, the Australian John Cade discovered that lithium salts could control mania, reducing the frequency and severity of manic episodes. This introduced the now popular drug lithium carbonate to the mainstream public, as well as being the first mood stabilizer to be approved by the U.S. Food & Drug Administration. Besides lithium, several anticonvulsants and atypical antipsychotics have mood stabilizing activity. The mechanism of action of mood stabilizers is not well understood.

Common mood stabilizers:

- Lithium (Lithobid, Eskalith), the oldest mood stabilizer.
- Carbamazepine (Tegretol), anticonvulsant and mood stabilizer.
- Oxcarbazepine (Trileptal), anticonvulsant and mood stabilizer.
- Valproic acid, and salts (Depakine, Depakote), anticonvulsant and mood stabilizer.
- Lamotrigine (Lamictal), atypical anticonvulsant and mood stabilizer.
- Gabapentin, atypical GABA-related anticonvulsant and mood stabilizer.
- Pregabalin, atypical GABA-ergic anticonvulsant and mood stabilizer.
- Topiramate, GABA-receptor related anticonvulsant and mood-stabilizer.
- Quetiapine, atypical antipsychotic and mood stabilizer.

Stimulants

A stimulant is a drug that stimulates the central nervous system, increasing arousal, attention and endurance. Stimulants are used in psychiatry to treat attention deficit-hyperactivity disorder. Because the medications can be addictive, patients with a history of drug abuse are typically monitored closely or treated with a non-stimulant.

Common Stimulants

- Methylphenidate (Ritalin, Concerta), a norepinephrine-dopamine reuptake inhibitor.
- Dexmethylphenidate (Focalin), the active dextro-enantiomer of methylphenidate.
- Mixed amphetamine salts (Adderall), a 3:1 mix of dextro/levo-enantiomers of amphetamine.
- Dextroamphetamine (Dexedrine), the dextro-enantiomer of amphetamine.
- Lisdexamfetamine (Vyvanse), a prodrug containing the dextro-enantiomer of amphetamine.

- Methamphetamine (Desoxyn), a potent but infrequently prescribed amphetamine.

Benzodiazepine

Benzodiazepines (BZD, BDZ, BZs), sometimes called "benzos", are a class of psychoactive drugs whose core chemical structure is the fusion of a benzene ring and a diazepine ring. The first such drug, chlordiazepoxide (Librium), was discovered accidentally by Leo Sternbach in 1955, and made available in 1960 by Hoffmann–La Roche, which, since 1963, has also marketed the benzodiazepine diazepam (Valium). In 1977 benzodiazepines were globally the most prescribed medications. They are in the family of drugs commonly known as minor tranquilizers.

Benzodiazepines enhance the effect of the neurotransmitter gamma-aminobutyric acid (GABA) at the $GABA_A$ receptor, resulting in sedative, hypnotic (sleep-inducing), anxiolytic (anti-anxiety), anticonvulsant, and muscle relaxant properties. High doses of many shorter-acting benzodiazepines may also cause anterograde amnesia and dissociation. These properties make benzodiazepines useful in treating anxiety, insomnia, agitation, seizures, muscle spasms, alcohol withdrawal and as a premedication for medical or dental procedures. Benzodiazepines are categorized as either short, intermediary, or long-acting. Short- and intermediate-acting benzodiazepines are preferred for the treatment of insomnia; longer-acting benzodiazepines are recommended for the treatment of anxiety.

Benzodiazepines are generally viewed as safe and effective for short-term use, although cognitive impairment and paradoxical effects such as aggression or behavioral disinhibition occasionally occur. A minority of people can have paradoxical reactions such as worsened agitation or panic. Benzodiazepines are also associated with increased risk of suicide. Long-term use is controversial because of concerns about decreasing effectiveness, physical dependence, withdrawal, and an increased risk of dementia. Stopping benzodiazepines often leads to improved physical and mental health. The elderly are at an increased risk of both short- and long-term adverse effects, and as a result, all benzodiazepines are listed in the Beers List of inappropriate medications for older adults. There is controversy concerning the safety of benzodiazepines in pregnancy. While they are not major teratogens, uncertainty remains as to whether they cause cleft palate in a small number of babies and whether neurobehavioural effects occur as a result of prenatal exposure; they are known to cause withdrawal symptoms in the newborn.

Benzodiazepines can be taken in overdoses and can cause dangerous deep unconsciousness. However, they are less toxic than their predecessors, the barbiturates, and death rarely results when a benzodiazepine is the only drug taken. When combined with other central nervous system (CNS) depressants such as alcoholic drinks and opioids, the potential for toxicity and fatal overdose increases. Benzodiazepines are commonly misused and taken in combination with other drugs of abuse.

Medical Uses

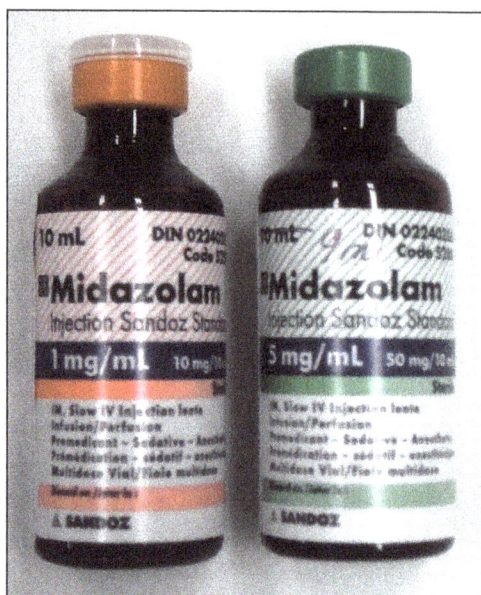

Midazolam 1 & 5 mg/mL injections.

Benzodiazepines possess psycholeptic, sedative, hypnotic, anxiolytic, anticonvulsant, muscle relaxant, and amnesic actions, which are useful in a variety of indications such as alcohol dependence, seizures, anxiety disorders, panic, agitation, and insomnia. Most are administered orally; however, they can also be given intravenously, intramuscularly, or rectally. In general, benzodiazepines are well-tolerated and are safe and effective drugs in the short term for a wide range of conditions. Tolerance can develop to their effects and there is also a risk of dependence, and upon discontinuation a withdrawal syndrome may occur. These factors, combined with other possible secondary effects after prolonged use such as psychomotor, cognitive, or memory impairments, limit their long-term applicability. The effects of long-term use or misuse include the tendency to cause or worsen cognitive deficits, depression, and anxiety. The College of Physicians and Surgeons of British Columbia recommends discontinuing the usage of benzodiazepines in those on opioids and those who have used them long term. Benzodiazepines can have serious adverse health outcomes, and these findings support clinical and regulatory efforts to reduce usage, especially in combination with non-benzodiazepine receptor agonists.

Panic Disorder

Because of their effectiveness, tolerability, and rapid onset of anxiolytic action, benzodiazepines are frequently used for the treatment of anxiety associated with panic disorder. However, there is disagreement among expert bodies regarding the long-term use of benzodiazepines for panic disorder. The views range from those that hold that benzodiazepines are not effective long-term and that they should be reserved for treatment-resistant cases to those that hold that they are as effective in the long term as selective serotonin reuptake inhibitors.

In general, benzodiazepines are well tolerated, and their use for the initial treatment for panic disorder is strongly supported by numerous controlled trials. APA states that there is insufficient evidence to recommend any of the established panic disorder treatments over another. The choice of treatment between benzodiazepines, SSRIs, serotonin–norepinephrine reuptake inhibitors, tricyclic antidepressants, and psychotherapy should be based on the patient's history, preference, and other individual characteristics. Selective serotonin reuptake inhibitors are likely to be the best choice of pharmacotherapy for many patients with panic disorder, but benzodiazepines are also often used, and some studies suggest that these medications are still used with greater frequency than the SSRIs. One advantage of benzodiazepines is that they alleviate the anxiety symptoms much faster than antidepressants, and therefore may be preferred in patients for whom rapid symptom control is critical. However, this advantage is offset by the possibility of developing benzodiazepine dependence. APA does not recommend benzodiazepines for persons with depressive symptoms or a recent history of substance abuse. The APA guidelines state that, in general, pharmacotherapy of panic disorder should be continued for at least a year, and that clinical experience supports continuing benzodiazepine treatment to prevent recurrence. Although major concerns about benzodiazepine tolerance and withdrawal have been raised, there is no evidence for significant dose escalation in patients using benzodiazepines long-term. For many such patients, stable doses of benzodiazepines retain their efficacy over several years.

Guidelines issued by the UK-based National Institute for Health and Clinical Excellence (NICE), carried out a systematic review using different methodology and came to a different conclusion. They questioned the accuracy of studies that were not placebo-controlled. And, based on the findings of placebo-controlled studies, they do not recommend use of benzodiazepines beyond two to four weeks, as tolerance and physical dependence develop rapidly, with withdrawal symptoms including rebound anxiety occurring after six weeks or more of use. Nevertheless, benzodiazepines are still prescribed for long-term treatment of anxiety disorders, although specific antidepressants and psychological therapies are recommended as the first-line treatment options with the anticonvulsant drug pregabalin indicated as a second- or third-line treatment and suitable for long-term use. NICE stated that long-term use of benzodiazepines for panic disorder with or without agoraphobia is an unlicensed indication, does not have long-term efficacy, and is, therefore, not recommended by clinical guidelines. Psychological therapies such as cognitive behavioural therapy are recommended as a first-line therapy for panic disorder; benzodiazepine use has been found to interfere with therapeutic gains from these therapies.

Benzodiazepines are usually administered orally; however, very occasionally lorazepam or diazepam may be given intravenously for the treatment of panic attacks.

Generalized Anxiety Disorder

Benzodiazepines have robust efficacy in the short-term management of generalized anxiety disorder (GAD), but were not shown effective in producing long-term improvement overall. According to National Institute for Health and Clinical Excellence (NICE), benzodiazepines can be used in the immediate management of GAD, if necessary. However, they should not usually be given for longer than 2–4 weeks. The only medications NICE recommends for the longer term management of GAD are antidepressants.

Likewise, Canadian Psychiatric Association (CPA) recommends benzodiazepines alprazolam, bromazepam, lorazepam, and diazepam only as a second-line choice, if the treatment with two different antidepressants was unsuccessful. Although they are second-line agents, benzodiazepines can be used for a limited time to relieve severe anxiety and agitation. CPA guidelines note that after 4–6 weeks the effect of benzodiazepines may decrease to the level of placebo, and that benzodiazepines are less effective than antidepressants in alleviating ruminative worry, the core symptom of GAD. However, in some cases, a prolonged treatment with benzodiazepines as the add-on to an antidepressant may be justified.

A 2015 review found a larger effect with medications than talk therapy. Medications with benefit include serotonin-noradrenaline reuptake inhibitors, benzodiazepines, and selective serotonin reuptake inhibitors.

Insomnia

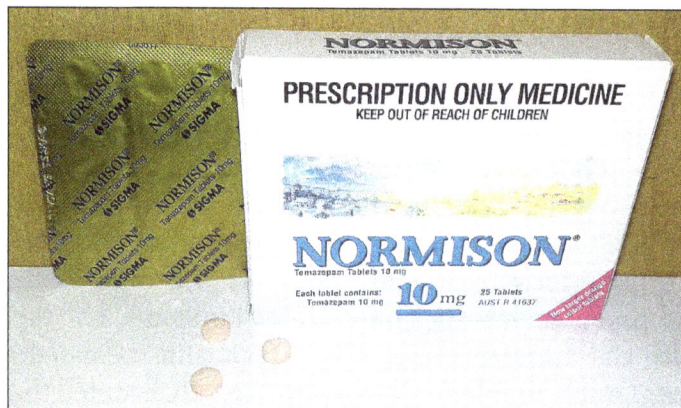

Temazepam (Normison) 10 mg tablets.

Benzodiazepines can be useful for short-term treatment of insomnia. Their use beyond 2 to 4 weeks is not recommended due to the risk of dependence. The Committee on Safety of Medicines report recommended that where long-term use of benzodiazepines for insomnia is indicated then treatment should be intermittent wherever possible. It is preferred that benzodiazepines be taken intermittently and at the lowest effective dose. They improve sleep-related problems by shortening the time spent in bed before falling asleep, prolonging the sleep time, and, in general, reducing wakefulness. However, they worsen sleep quality by increasing light sleep and decreasing deep sleep. Other drawbacks of hypnotics, including benzodiazepines, are possible tolerance to their effects, rebound insomnia, and reduced slow-wave sleep and a withdrawal period typified by rebound insomnia and a prolonged period of anxiety and agitation.

The list of benzodiazepines approved for the treatment of insomnia is fairly similar among most countries, but which benzodiazepines are officially designated as first-line hypnotics prescribed for the treatment of insomnia varies between countries. Longer-acting benzodiazepines such as nitrazepam and diazepam have residual effects that may persist into the next day and are, in general, not recommended.

Since the release of non benzodiazepines in 1992 in response to safety concerns, individuals with insomnia and other sleep disorders have increasingly been prescribed nonbenzodiazepines (2.3% in 1993 to 13.7% of Americans in 2010), less often prescribed benzodiazepines (23.5% in 1993 to 10.8% in 2010). It is not clear as to whether the new non benzodiazepine hypnotics (Z-drugs) are better than the short-acting benzodiazepines. The efficacy of these two groups of medications is similar. According to the US Agency for Healthcare Research and Quality, indirect comparison indicates that side-effects from benzodiazepines may be about twice as frequent as from nonbenzodiazepines. Some experts suggest using nonbenzodiazepines preferentially as a first-line long-term treatment of insomnia. However, the UK National Institute for Health and Clinical Excellence did not find any convincing evidence in favor of Z-drugs. NICE review pointed out that short-acting Z-drugs were inappropriately compared in clinical trials with long-acting benzodiazepines. There have been no trials comparing short-acting Z-drugs with appropriate doses of short-acting benzodiazepines. Based on this, NICE recommended choosing the hypnotic based on cost and the patient's preference.

Older adults should not use benzodiazepines to treat insomnia unless other treatments have failed. When benzodiazepines are used, patients, their caretakers, and their physician should discuss the increased risk of harms, including evidence that shows twice the incidence of traffic collisions among driving patients, and falls and hip fracture for older patients.

Seizures

Prolonged convulsive epileptic seizures are a medical emergency that can usually be dealt with effectively by administering fast-acting benzodiazepines, which are potent anticonvulsants. In a hospital environment, intravenous clonazepam, lorazepam, and diazepam are first-line choices. In the community, intravenous administration is not practical and so rectal diazepam or buccal midazolam are used, with a preference for midazolam as its administration is easier and more socially acceptable.

When benzodiazepines were first introduced, they were enthusiastically adopted for treating all forms of epilepsy. However, drowsiness and tolerance become problems with continued use and none are now considered first-line choices for long-term epilepsy therapy. Clobazam is widely used by specialist epilepsy clinics worldwide and clonazepam is popular in the Netherlands, Belgium and France. Clobazam was approved for use in the United States in 2011. In the UK, both clobazam and clonazepam are second-line choices for treating many forms of epilepsy. Clobazam also has a useful role for very short-term seizure prophylaxis and in catamenial epilepsy. Discontinuation after long-term use in epilepsy requires additional caution because of the risks of rebound seizures. Therefore, the dose is slowly tapered over a period of up to six months or longer.

Alcohol Withdrawal

Chlordiazepoxide is the most commonly used benzodiazepine for alcohol detoxification, but diazepam may be used as an alternative. Both are used in the detoxification of individuals who are motivated to stop drinking, and are prescribed for a short period of time to reduce the risks of developing tolerance and dependence to the benzodiazepine medication itself. The benzodiazepines with a longer half-life make detoxification more tolerable, and dangerous (and potentially lethal) alcohol withdrawal effects are less likely to occur. On the other hand, short-acting benzodiazepines may lead to breakthrough seizures, and are, therefore, not recommended for detoxification in an outpatient setting. Oxazepam and lorazepam are often used in patients at risk of drug accumulation, in particular, the elderly and those with cirrhosis, because they are metabolized differently from other benzodiazepines, through conjugation.

Benzodiazepines are the preferred choice in the management of alcohol withdrawal syndrome, in particular, for the prevention and treatment of the dangerous complication of seizures and in subduing severe delirium. Lorazepam is the only benzodiazepine with predictable intramuscular absorption and it is the most effective in preventing and controlling acute seizures.

Anxiety

Benzodiazepines are sometimes used in the treatment of acute anxiety, as they bring about rapid and marked or moderate relief of symptoms in most individuals; however, they are not recommended beyond 2–4 weeks of use due to risks of tolerance and dependence and a lack of long-term effectiveness. As for insomnia, they may also be used on an irregular/"as-needed" basis, such as in cases where said anxiety is at its worst. Compared to other pharmacological treatments, benzodiazepines are twice as likely to lead to a relapse of the underlying condition upon discontinuation. Psychological therapies and other pharmacological therapies are recommended for the long-term treatment of generalized anxiety disorder. Antidepressants have higher remission rates and are, in general, safe and effective in the short and long term.

Other Indications

Benzodiazepines are often prescribed for a wide range of conditions:

- They can sedate patients receiving mechanical ventilation or those in extreme distress. Caution is exercised in this situation due to the risk of respiratory depression, and it is recommended that benzodiazepine overdose treatment facilities should be available.

- Benzodiazepines are indicated in the management of breathlessness (shortness of breath) in advanced diseases, in particular where other treatments have failed to adequately control symptoms.

- Benzodiazepines are effective as medication given a couple of hours before surgery to relieve anxiety. They also produce amnesia, which can be useful, as patients may not remember unpleasantness from the procedure. They are also used in patients with dental phobia as well as some ophthalmic procedures like refractive surgery; although such use is controversial and only recommended for those who are very anxious. Midazolam is the most commonly prescribed for this use because of its strong sedative actions and fast recovery time, as well as its water solubility, which reduces pain upon injection. Diazepam and lorazepam are sometimes used. Lorazepam has particularly marked amnesic properties that may make it more effective when amnesia is the desired effect.

- Benzodiazepines are well known for their strong muscle-relaxing properties and can be useful in the treatment of muscle spasms, although tolerance often develops to their muscle relaxant effects. Baclofen or tizanidine are sometimes used as an alternative to benzodiazepines. Tizanidine has been found to have superior tolerability compared to diazepam and baclofen.

- Benzodiazepines are also used to treat the acute panic caused by hallucinogen intoxication. Benzodiazepines are also used to calm the acutely agitated individual and can, if required, be given via an intramuscular injection. They can sometimes be effective in the short-term treatment of psychiatric emergencies such as acute psychosis as in schizophrenia or mania, bringing about rapid tranquillization and sedation until the effects of lithium or neuroleptics (antipsychotics) take effect. Lorazepam is most commonly used but clonazepam is sometimes prescribed for acute psychosis or mania; their long-term use is not recommended due to risks of dependence. Further research investigating the use of benzodiazepines alone and in combination with antipsychotic medications for treating acute psychosis is warranted.

- Clonazepam, a benzodiazepine is used to treat many forms of parasomnia. Rapid eye movement behavior disorder responds well to low doses of clonazepam. Restless legs syndrome can be treated using clonazepam as a third line treatment option as the use of clonazepam is still investigational.

- Benzodiazepines are sometimes used for obsessive–compulsive disorder (OCD), although they are generally believed ineffective for this indication. Effectiveness was, however, found in one small study. Benzodiazepines can be considered as a treatment option in treatment resistant cases.

- Antipsychotics are generally a first-line treatment for delirium; however, when delirium is caused by alcohol or sedative hypnotic withdrawal, benzodiazepines are a first-line treatment.

- There is some evidence that low doses of benzodiazepines reduce adverse effects of electroconvulsive therapy.

Contraindications

Because of their muscle relaxant action, benzodiazepines may cause respiratory depression in susceptible individuals. For that reason, they are contraindicated in people with myasthenia gravis, sleep apnea, bronchitis, and COPD. Caution is required when benzodiazepines are used in people with personality disorders or intellectual disability because of frequent paradoxical reactions. In major depression, they may precipitate suicidal tendencies and are sometimes used for suicidal overdoses. Individuals with a history of alcohol, opioid and barbiturate abuse should avoid benzodiazepines, as there is a risk of life-threatening interactions with these drugs.

Pregnancy

In the United States, the Food and Drug Administration has categorized benzodiazepines into either category D or X meaning potential for harm in the unborn has been demonstrated.

Exposure to benzodiazepines during pregnancy has been associated with a slightly increased (from 0.06 to 0.07%) risk of cleft palate in newborns, a controversial conclusion as some studies find no association between benzodiazepines and cleft palate. Their use by expectant mothers shortly before the delivery may result in a floppy infant syndrome, with the newborns suffering from hypotonia, hypothermia, lethargy, and breathing and feeding difficulties. Cases of neonatal withdrawal syndrome have been described in infants chronically exposed to benzodiazepines in utero. This syndrome may be hard to recognize, as it starts several days after delivery, for example, as late as 21 days for chlordiazepoxide. The symptoms include tremors, hypertonia, hyperreflexia, hyperactivity, and vomiting and may last for up to three to six months. Tapering down the dose during pregnancy may lessen its severity. If used in pregnancy, those benzodiazepines with a better and longer safety record, such as diazepam or chlordiazepoxide, are recommended over potentially more harmful benzodiazepines, such as temazepam or triazolam. Using the lowest effective dose for the shortest period of time minimizes the risks to the unborn child.

Elderly

The benefits of benzodiazepines are least and the risks are greatest in the elderly. They are listed as a potentially inappropriate medication for older adults by the American Geriatrics Society. The elderly are at an increased risk of dependence and are more sensitive to the adverse effects such as memory problems, daytime sedation, impaired motor coordination, and increased risk of motor vehicle accidents and falls, and an increased risk of hip fractures. The long-term effects of benzodiazepines and benzodiazepine dependence in the elderly can resemble dementia, depression, or anxiety syndromes, and progressively worsens over time. Adverse effects on cognition can be mistaken for the effects of old age. The benefits of withdrawal include improved cognition, alertness, mobility, reduced risk incontinence, and a reduced risk of falls and fractures. The success of gradual-tapering benzodiazepines is as great in the elderly as in younger people. Benzodiazepines should be prescribed to the elderly only with caution and only for a short period at low doses. Short to intermediate-acting benzodiazepines are preferred in the elderly such as oxazepam and temazepam. The high potency benzodiazepines alprazolam and triazolam and long-acting benzodiazepines are not recommended in the elderly due to increased adverse effects. Nonbenzodiazepines such as zaleplon and zolpidem and low doses of sedating antidepressants are sometimes used as alternatives to benzodiazepines.

Long-term use of benzodiazepines is associated with increased risk of cognitive impairment and dementia, and reduction in prescribing levels is likely to reduce dementia risk. The association of a past history of benzodiazepine use and cognitive decline is unclear, with some studies reporting a lower risk of cognitive decline in former users, some finding no association and some indicating an increased risk of cognitive decline.

Benzodiazepines are sometimes prescribed to treat behavioral symptoms of dementia. However, like antidepressants, they have little evidence of effectiveness, although antipsychotics have shown some benefit. Cognitive impairing effects of benzodiazepines that occur frequently in the elderly can also worsen dementia.

Adverse Effects

The most common side-effects of benzodiazepines are related to their sedating and muscle-relaxing action. They include drowsiness, dizziness, and decreased alertness and concentration. Lack of coordination may result in falls and injuries, in particular, in the elderly. Another result is impairment of driving skills and increased likelihood of road traffic accidents. Decreased libido and erection problems are a common side effect. Depression and disinhibition may emerge. Hypotension and suppressed breathing (hypoventilation) may be encountered with intravenous use. Less common side effects include nausea and changes in appetite, blurred vision, confusion, euphoria, depersonalization and nightmares. Cases of liver toxicity have been described but are very rare.

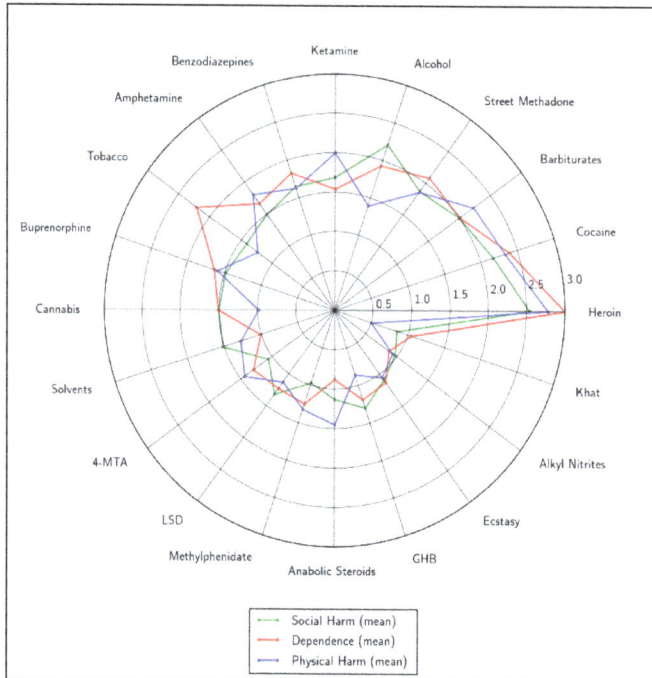

Addiction experts in psychiatry, chemistry, pharmacology, forensic science, epidemiology,
and the police and legal services engaged in delphic analysis regarding 20 popular recreational drugs.
Benzodiazepines were ranked in this graph 7th in dependence, physical harm, and social harm.

The long-term effects of benzodiazepine use can include cognitive impairment as well as
affective and behavioural problems. Feelings of turmoil, difficulty in thinking construc-
tively, loss of sex-drive, agoraphobia and social phobia, increasing anxiety and depression, loss of interest in leisure pursuits and interests, and an inability to experience or
express feelings can also occur. Not everyone, however, experiences problems with long-
term use. Additionally, an altered perception of self, environment and relationships may
occur.

Compared to other sedative-hypnotics, visits to the hospital involving benzodiazepines
had a 66% greater odds of a serious adverse health outcome. This included hospitalization, patient transfer, or death, and visits involving a combination of benzodiazepines
and non-benzodiapine receptor agonists had almost four-times increased odds of a serious health outcome.

Cognitive Effects

The short-term use of benzodiazepines adversely affects multiple areas of cognition,
the most notable one being that it interferes with the formation and consolidation of
memories of new material and may induce complete anterograde amnesia. However,
researchers hold contrary opinions regarding the effects of long-term administration.
One view is that many of the short-term effects continue into the long-term and may
even worsen, and are not resolved after stopping benzodiazepine usage. Another view

maintains that cognitive deficits in chronic benzodiazepine users occur only for a short period after the dose, or that the anxiety disorder is the cause of these deficits.

While the definitive studies are lacking, the former view received support from a 2004 meta-analysis of 13 small studies. This meta-analysis found that long-term use of benzodiazepines was associated with moderate to large adverse effects on all areas of cognition, with visuospatial memory being the most commonly detected impairment. Some of the other impairments reported were decreased IQ, visiomotor coordination, information processing, verbal learning and concentration. The authors of the meta-analysis and a later reviewer noted that the applicability of this meta-analysis is limited because the subjects were taken mostly from withdrawal clinics; the coexisting drug, alcohol use, and psychiatric disorders were not defined; and several of the included studies conducted the cognitive measurements during the withdrawal period.

Paradoxical Effects

Paradoxical reactions, such as increased seizures in epileptics, aggression, violence, impulsivity, irritability and suicidal behavior sometimes occur. These reactions have been explained as consequences of disinhibition and the subsequent loss of control over socially unacceptable behavior. Paradoxical reactions are rare in the general population, with an incidence rate below 1% and similar to placebo. However, they occur with greater frequency in recreational abusers, individuals with borderline personality disorder, children, and patients on high-dosage regimes. In these groups, impulse control problems are perhaps the most important risk factor for disinhibition; learning disabilities and neurological disorders are also significant risks. Most reports of disinhibition involve high doses of high-potency benzodiazepines. Paradoxical effects may also appear after chronic use of benzodiazepines.

Long-term Worsening of Psychiatric Symptoms

While benzodiazepines may have short-term benefits for anxiety, sleep and agitation in some patients, long-term (i.e. greater than 2–4 weeks) use can result in a worsening of the very symptoms the medications are meant to treat. Potential explanations include exacerbating cognitive problems that are already common in anxiety disorders, causing or worsening depression and suicidality, disrupting sleep architecture by inhibiting deep stage sleep, withdrawal symptoms or rebound symptoms in between doses mimicking or exacerbating underlying anxiety or sleep disorders, inhibiting the benefits of psychotherapy by inhibiting memory consolidation and reducing fear extinction, and reducing coping with trauma/stress and increasing vulnerability to future stress. Anxiety, insomnia and irritability may be temporarily exacerbated during withdrawal, but psychiatric symptoms after discontinuation are usually less than even while taking benzodiazepines. Functioning significantly improves within 1 year of discontinuation.

Reinforcement Disorders

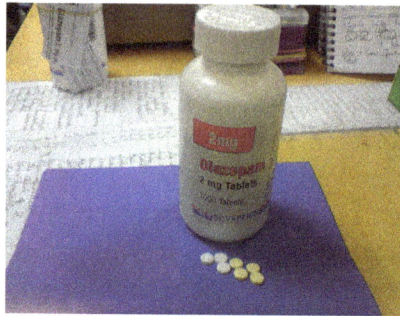

Diazepam 2 mg and 5 mg diazepam tablets, which are commonly used
in the treatment of benzodiazepine withdrawal.

Tolerance

The main problem of the chronic use of benzodiazepines is the development of tolerance and dependence. Tolerance manifests itself as diminished pharmacological effect and develops relatively quickly to the sedative, hypnotic, anticonvulsant, and muscle relaxant actions of benzodiazepines. Tolerance to anti-anxiety effects develops more slowly with little evidence of continued effectiveness beyond four to six months of continued use. In general, tolerance to the amnesic effects does not occur. However, controversy exists as to tolerance to the anxiolytic effects with some evidence that benzodiazepines retain efficacy and opposing evidence from a systematic review of the literature that tolerance frequently occurs and some evidence that anxiety may worsen with long-term use. The question of tolerance to the amnesic effects of benzodiazepines is, likewise, unclear. Some evidence suggests that partial tolerance does develop, and that, "memory impairment is limited to a narrow window within 90 minutes after each dose".

A major disadvantage of benzodiazepines that tolerance to therapeutic effects develops relatively quickly while many adverse effects persist. Tolerance develops to hypnotic and myorelaxant effects within days to weeks, and to anticonvulsant and anxiolytic effects within weeks to months. Therefore, benzodiazepines are unlikely to be effective long-term treatments for sleep and anxiety. While BZD therapeutic effects disappear with tolerance, depression and impulsivity with high suicidal risk commonly persist. Several studies have confirmed that long-term benzodiazepines are not significantly different from placebo for sleep or anxiety. This may explain why patients commonly increase doses over time and many eventually take more than one type of benzodiazepine after the first loses effectiveness. Additionally, because tolerance to benzodiazepine sedating effects develops more quickly than does tolerance to brainstem depressant effects, those taking more benzodiazepines to achieve desired effects may suffer sudden respiratory depression, hypotension or death. Most patients with anxiety disorders and PTSD have symptoms that persist for at least several months, making tolerance to therapeutic effects a distinct problem for them and necessitating the need for more effective long-term treatment (e.g. psychotherapy, serotonergic antidepressants).

Withdrawal Symptoms and Management

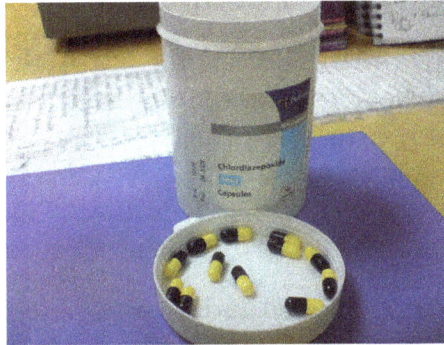

Chlordiazepoxide 5 mg capsules, which are sometimes used as an alternative to
diazepam for benzodiazepine withdrawal. Like diazepam it has a long
elimination half-life and long-acting active metabolites.

Discontinuation of benzodiazepines or abrupt reduction of the dose, even after a
relatively short course of treatment (two to four weeks), may result in two groups of
symptoms—rebound and withdrawal. Rebound symptoms are the return of the symptoms for which the patient was treated but worse than before. Withdrawal symptoms
are the new symptoms that occur when the benzodiazepine is stopped. They are the
main sign of physical dependence.

The most frequent symptoms of withdrawal from benzodiazepines are insomnia, gastric problems, tremors, agitation, fearfulness, and muscle spasms. The less frequent
effects are irritability, sweating, depersonalization, derealization, hypersensitivity to
stimuli, depression, suicidal behavior, psychosis, seizures, and delirium tremens. Severe symptoms usually occur as a result of abrupt or over-rapid withdrawal. Abrupt
withdrawal can be dangerous, therefore a gradual reduction regimen is recommended.

Symptoms may also occur during a gradual dosage reduction, but are typically less
severe and may persist as part of a protracted withdrawal syndrome for months after cessation of benzodiazepines. Approximately 10% of patients experience a notable
protracted withdrawal syndrome, which can persist for many months or in some cases
a year or longer. Protracted symptoms tend to resemble those seen during the first
couple of months of withdrawal but usually are of a sub-acute level of severity. Such
symptoms do gradually lessen over time, eventually disappearing altogether.

Benzodiazepines have a reputation with patients and doctors for causing a severe and
traumatic withdrawal; however, this is in large part due to the withdrawal process being poorly managed. Over-rapid withdrawal from benzodiazepines increases the severity of the withdrawal syndrome and increases the failure rate. A slow and gradual withdrawal customised to the individual and, if indicated, psychological support is the most
effective way of managing the withdrawal. Opinion as to the time needed to complete
withdrawal ranges from four weeks to several years. A goal of less than six months has
been suggested, but due to factors such as dosage and type of benzodiazepine, reasons

for prescription, lifestyle, personality, environmental stresses, and amount of available support, a year or more may be needed to withdraw.

Withdrawal is best managed by transferring the physically dependent patient to an equivalent dose of diazepam because it has the longest half-life of all of the benzodiazepines, is metabolised into long-acting active metabolites and is available in low-potency tablets, which can be quartered for smaller doses. A further benefit is that it is available in liquid form, which allows for even smaller reductions. Chlordiazepoxide, which also has a long half-life and long-acting active metabolites, can be used as an alternative.

Nonbenzodiazepines are contraindicated during benzodiazepine withdrawal as they are cross tolerant with benzodiazepines and can induce dependence. Alcohol is also cross tolerant with benzodiazepines and more toxic and thus caution is needed to avoid replacing one dependence with another. During withdrawal, fluoroquinolone-based antibiotics are best avoided if possible; they displace benzodiazepines from their binding site and reduce GABA function and, thus, may aggravate withdrawal symptoms. Antipsychotics are not recommended for benzodiazepine withdrawal (or other CNS depressant withdrawal states) especially clozapine, olanzapine or low potency phenothiazines e.g. chlorpromazine as they lower the seizure threshold and can worsen withdrawal effects; if used extreme caution is required.

Withdrawal from long term benzodiazepines is beneficial for most individuals. Withdrawal of benzodiazepines from long-term users, in general, leads to improved physical and mental health particularly in the elderly; although some long term users report continued benefit from taking benzodiazepines, this may be the result of suppression of withdrawal effects.

Controversial Associations

Beyond the well established link between benzodiazepines and psychomotor impairment resulting in motor vehicle accidents and falls leading to fracture; research in the 2000s and 2010s has raised the association between benzodiazepines (and Z-Drugs) and other, as of yet unproven, adverse effects including dementia, cancer, infections, pancreatitis and respiratory disease exacerbations.

Dementia

A number of studies have drawn an association between long-term benzodiazepine use and neuro-degenerative disease, particularly Alzheimer's disease. It has been determined that long-term use of benzodiazepines is associated with increased dementia risk, even after controlling for protopathic bias.

Infections

Some observational studies have detected significant associations between benzodiazepines and respiratory infections such as pneumonia where others have not. A large meta-analysis of pre-marketing randomized controlled trials on the pharmacologically related Z-Drugs suggest a small increase in infection risk as well. An immunodeficiency effect from the action of benzodiazepines on GABA-A receptors has been postulated from animal studies.

Cancer

A Meta-analysis of observational studies has determined an association between benzodiazepine use and cancer, though the risk across different agents and different cancers varied significantly. Furthermore, most of these studies were unable to control for confounding variables that may have influenced the relationship such as lifestyle exposures (i.e. tobacco, alcohol). In terms of experimental basic science evidence, an analysis of carcinogenetic and genotoxicity data for various benzodiazepines has suggested a small possibility of carcinogenesis for a small number of benzodiazepines. A large, properly designed randomized controlled trial with appropriate follow-up in addition to further pharmacologic/toxicologic investigation is needed to confirm these preliminary findings.

Pancreatitis

The evidence suggesting a link between benzodiazepines (and Z-Drugs) and pancreatic inflammation is very sparse and limited to a few observational studies from Taiwan. A criticism of confounding can be applied to these findings as with the other controversial associations above. Further well-designed research from other populations as well as a biologically plausible mechanism is required to confirm this association.

Overdose

Although benzodiazepines are much safer in overdose than their predecessors, the barbiturates, they can still cause problems in overdose. Taken alone, they rarely cause severe complications in overdose; statistics in England showed that benzodiazepines were responsible for 3.8% of all deaths by poisoning from a single drug. However, combining these drugs with alcohol, opiates or tricyclic antidepressants markedly raises the toxicity. The elderly are more sensitive to the side effects of benzodiazepines, and poisoning may even occur from their long-term use. The various benzodiazepines differ in their toxicity; temazepam appears most toxic in overdose and when used with other drugs. The symptoms of a benzodiazepine overdose may include; drowsiness, slurred speech, nystagmus, hypotension, ataxia, coma, respiratory depression, and cardiorespiratory arrest.

A reversal agent for benzodiazepines exists, flumazenil (Anexate). Its use as an antidote is not routinely recommended because of the high risk of resedation and seizures. In a double-blind, placebo-controlled trial of 326 people, 4 people had serious adverse events and 61% became resedated following the use of flumazenil. Numerous contraindications to its use exist. It is contraindicated in people with a history of long-term use of benzodiazepines, those having ingested a substance that lowers the seizure threshold or may cause an arrhythmia, and in those with abnormal vital signs. One study found that only 10% of the people presenting with a benzodiazepine overdose are suitable candidates for treatment with flumazenil.

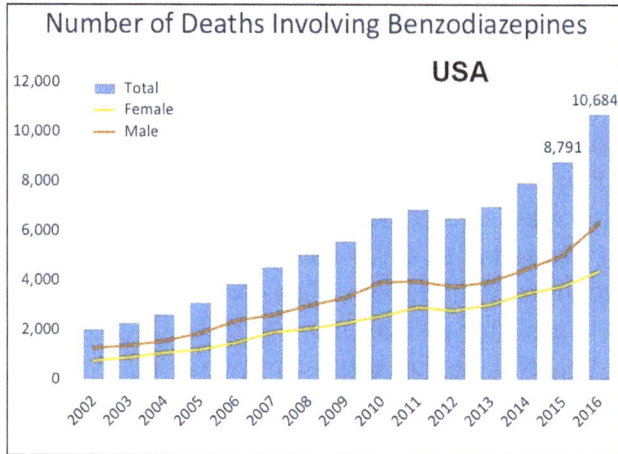

US yearly overdose deaths involving benzodiazepines.

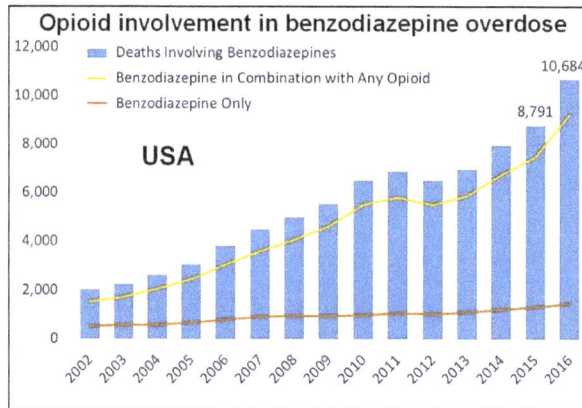

The top line represents the number of benzodiazepine deaths that also involved opioids in the US. The bottom line represents benzodiazepine deaths that did not involve opioids.

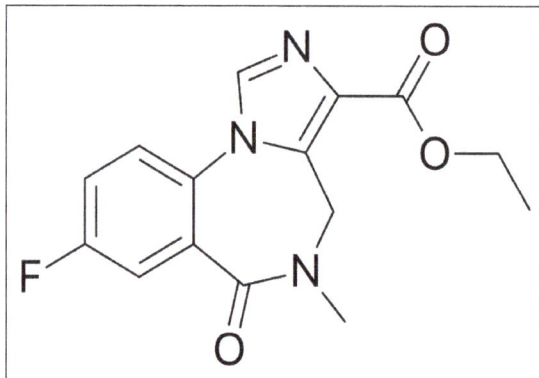

Chemical structure of the benzodiazepine flumazenil, whose use is controversial following benzodiazepine overdose.

Interactions

Individual benzodiazepines may have different interactions with certain drugs. Depending on their metabolism pathway, benzodiazepines can be divided roughly into two groups. The largest group consists of those that are metabolized by cytochrome P450 (CYP450) enzymes and possess significant potential for interactions with other drugs. The other group comprises those that are metabolized through glucuronidation, such as lorazepam, oxazepam, and temazepam, and, in general, have few drug interactions.

Many drugs, including oral contraceptives, some antibiotics, antidepressants, and antifungal agents, inhibit cytochrome enzymes in the liver. They reduce the rate of elimination of the benzodiazepines that are metabolized by CYP450, leading to possibly excessive drug accumulation and increased side-effects. In contrast, drugs that induce cytochrome P450 enzymes, such as St John's wort, the antibiotic rifampicin, and the anticonvulsants carbamazepine and phenytoin, accelerate elimination of many benzodiazepines and decrease their action. Taking benzodiazepines with alcohol, opioids and other central nervous system depressants potentiates their action. This often results in increased sedation, impaired motor coordination, suppressed breathing, and other adverse effects that have potential to be lethal. Antacids can slow down absorption of some benzodiazepines; however, this effect is marginal and inconsistent.

Pharmacodynamics

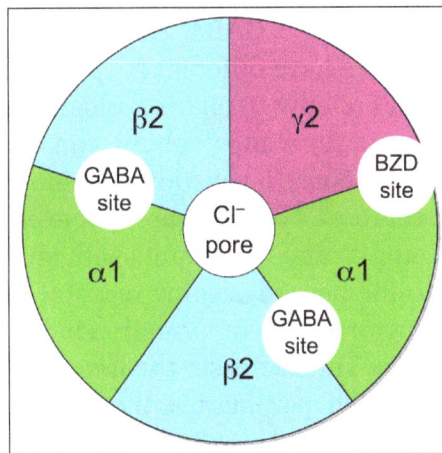

The above image is a schematic diagram of the $(\alpha 1)_2(\beta 2)_2(\gamma 2)$ GABA$_A$ receptor complex that depicts the five-protein subunits that form the receptor, the chloride (Cl$^-$) ion channel pore at the center, the two GABA| active binding sites at the $\alpha 1$ and $\beta 2$ interfaces and the benzodiazepine (BZD) allosteric binding site at the $\alpha 1$ and $\gamma 2$ interface.

Benzodiazepines work by increasing the effectiveness of the endogenous chemical, GABA, to decrease the excitability of neurons. This reduces the communication between neurons and, therefore, has a calming effect on many of the functions of the brain.

GABA controls the excitability of neurons by binding to the $GABA_A$ receptor. The GABA$_A$ receptor is a protein complex located in the synapses between neurons. All GABA$_A$ receptors contain an ion channel that conducts chloride ions across neuronal cell membranes and two binding sites for the neurotransmitter gamma-aminobutyric acid (GABA), while a subset of $GABA_A$ receptor complexes also contain a single binding site for benzodiazepines. Binding of benzodiazepines to this receptor complex does not alter binding of GABA. Unlike other positive allosteric modulators that increases ligand binding, benzodiazepine binding acts as a positive allosteric modulator by increasing the total conduction of chloride ions across the neuronal cell membrane when GABA is already bound to its receptor. This increased chloride ion influx hyperpolarizes the neuron's membrane potential. As a result, the difference between resting potential and threshold potential is increased and firing is less likely. Different $GABA_A$ receptor subtypes have varying distributions within different regions of the brain and, therefore, control distinct neuronal circuits. Hence, activation of different $GABA_A$ receptor subtypes by benzodiazepines may result in distinct pharmacological actions. In terms of the mechanism of action of benzodiazepines, their similarities are too great to separate them into individual categories such as anxiolytic or hypnotic. For example, a hypnotic administered in low doses produces anxiety-relieving effects, whereas a benzodiazepine marketed as an anti-anxiety drug at higher doses induces sleep.

The subset of $GABA_A$ receptors that also bind benzodiazepines are referred to as benzodiazepine receptors (BzR). The $GABA_A$ receptor is a heteromer composed of five subunits, the most common ones being two αs, two βs, and one γ ($\alpha_2\beta_2\gamma1$). For each subunit, many subtypes exist (α_{1-6}, β_{1-3}, and γ_{1-3}). $GABA_A$ receptors that are made up of different combinations of subunit subtypes have different properties, different distributions in the brain and different activities relative to pharmacological and clinical effects. Benzodiazepines bind at the interface of the α and γ subunits on the $GABA_A$ receptor. Binding also requires that alpha subunits contain a histidine amino acid residue, (i.e. α_1, α_2, α_3, and α_5 containing $GABA_A$ receptors). For this reason, benzodiazepines show no affinity for $GABA_A$ receptors containing α_4 and α_6 subunits with an arginine instead of a histidine residue. Once bound to the benzodiazepine receptor, the benzodiazepine ligand locks the benzodiazepine receptor into a conformation in which it has a greater affinity for the GABA neurotransmitter. This increases the frequency of the opening of the associated chloride ion channel and hyperpolarizes the membrane of the associated neuron. The inhibitory effect of the available GABA is potentiated, leading to sedative and anxiolytic effects. For instance, those ligands with high activity at the α_1 are associated with stronger hypnotic effects, whereas those with higher affinity for $GABA_A$ receptors containing α_2 and/or α_3 subunits have good anti-anxiety activity.

The benzodiazepine class of drugs also interact with peripheral benzodiazepine receptors. Peripheral benzodiazepine receptors are present in peripheral nervous system tissues, glial cells, and to a lesser extent the central nervous system. These peripheral receptors are not structurally related or coupled to $GABA_A$ receptors. They modulate the immune system and are involved in the body response to injury. Benzodiazepines also function as weak adenosine reuptake inhibitors. It has been suggested that some of their anticonvulsant, anxiolytic, and muscle relaxant effects may be in part mediated by this action. It also should be noted Benzodiazepines have binding sites in the periphery, however their effects on muscle tone is not mediated through these peripheral receptors. The peripheral binding sites for benzodiazepines are present in immune cells and gastrointestinal tract.

Pharmacokinetics

Benzodiazepine	Half-life (range, hours)	Speed of Onset
Alprazolam	6–15	Intermediate
Flunitrazepam	18-26	Fast
Chlordiazepoxide	10–30	Intermediate
Clonazepam	19–60	Slow
Diazepam	20–80	Fast
Lorazepam	10–20	Intermediate
Midazolam	1.5-2.5	Fast
Oxazepam	5–10	Slow
Prazepam	50–200	Slow

A benzodiazepine can be placed into one of three groups by its elimination half-life, or time it takes for the body to eliminate half of the dose. Some benzodiazepines have long-acting active metabolites, such as diazepam and chlordiazepoxide, which are metabolised into desmethyldiazepam. Desmethyldiazepam has a half-life of 36–200 hours, and flurazepam, with the main active metabolite of desalkylflurazepam, with a half-life of 40–250 hours. These long-acting metabolites are partial agonists.

- Short-acting compounds have a median half-life of 1–12 hours. They have few residual effects if taken before bedtime, rebound insomnia may occur upon discontinuation, and they might cause daytime withdrawal symptoms such as next day rebound anxiety with prolonged usage. Examples are brotizolam, midazolam, and triazolam.

- Intermediate-acting compounds have a median half-life of 12–40 hours. They may have some residual effects in the first half of the day if used as a hypnotic. Rebound insomnia, however, is more common upon discontinuation of intermediate-acting benzodiazepines than longer-acting benzodiazepines. Examples are alprazolam, estazolam, flunitrazepam, clonazepam, lormetazepam, lorazepam, nitrazepam, and temazepam.

- Long-acting compounds have a half-life of 40–250 hours. They have a risk of accumulation in the elderly and in individuals with severely impaired liver function, but they have a reduced severity of rebound effects and withdrawal. Examples are diazepam, clorazepate, chlordiazepoxide, and flurazepam.

Chemistry

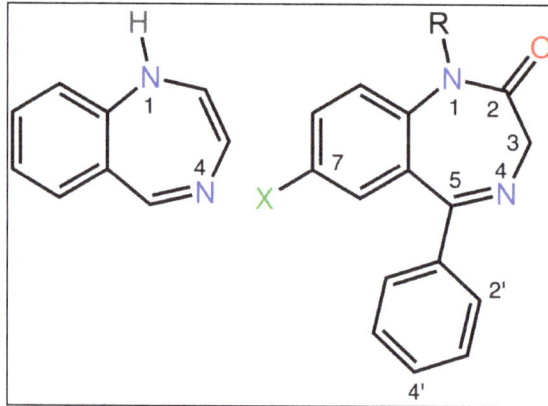

Top: The 1,4-benzodiazepine ring system. Bottom: 5-phenyl-1H-benzo[e] [1,4]diazepin-2(3H)-one forms the skeleton of many of the most common benzodiazepine pharmaceuticals, such as diazepam (7-chloro-1-methyl substituted).

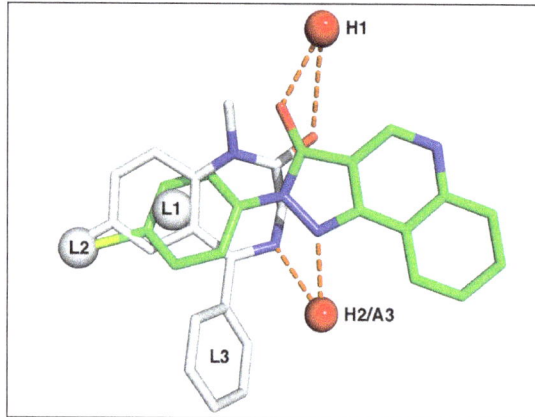

A pharmacophore model of the benzodiazepine binding site on the $GABA_A$ receptor. White sticks represent the carbon atoms of the benzodiazepine diazepam, while green represents carbon atoms of the nonbenzodiazepine CGS-9896. Red and blue sticks are oxygen and nitrogen atoms that are present in both structures. The red spheres labeled H1 and H2/A3 are, respectively, hydrogen bond donating and accepting sites in the receptor, while L1, L2, and L3 denote lipophilic binding sites.

Benzodiazepines share a similar chemical structure, and their effects in humans are mainly produced by the allosteric modification of a specific kind of neurotransmitter receptor, the $GABA_A$ receptor, which increases the overall conductance of these inhibitory channels; this results in the various therapeutic effects as well as adverse effects of benzodiazepines. Other less important modes of action are also known.

The term benzodiazepine is the chemical name for the heterocyclic ring system, which is a fusion between the benzene and diazepine ring systems. Under Hantzsch–Widman nomenclature, a diazepine is a heterocycle with two nitrogen atoms, five carbon atom and the maximum possible number of cumulative double bonds. The "benzo" prefix indicates the benzene ring fused onto the diazepine ring.

Benzodiazepine drugs are substituted 1,4-benzodiazepines, although the chemical term can refer to many other compounds that do not have useful pharmacological properties. Different benzodiazepine drugs have different side groups attached to this central structure. The different side groups affect the binding of the molecule to the GABA$_A$ receptor and so modulate the pharmacological properties. Many of the pharmacologically active "classical" benzodiazepine drugs contain the 5-phenyl-1H-benzo[e] [1,4]diazepin-2(3H)-one substructure. Benzodiazepines have been found to mimic protein reverse turns structurally, which enable them with their biological activity in many cases.

Nonbenzodiazepines also bind to the benzodiazepine binding site on the GABA$_A$ receptor and possess similar pharmacological properties. While the nonbenzodiazepines are by definition structurally unrelated to the benzodiazepines, both classes of drugs possess a common pharmacophore, which explains their binding to a common receptor site.

Common Types

- 2-keto compounds: Clorazepate, diazepam, flurazepam, halazepam, prazepam, and others.

- 3-hydroxy compounds: Lorazepam, lormetazepam, oxazepam, temazepam.

- 7-nitro compounds: Clonazepam, flunitrazepam, nimetazepam, nitrazepam.

- Triazolo compounds: Adinazolam, alprazolam, estazolam, triazolam.

- Imidazo compounds: Climazolam, loprazolam, midazolam.

Hallucinogen

A hallucinogen is a psychoactive agent which can cause hallucinations, perceptual anomalies, and other substantial subjective changes in thoughts, emotion, and consciousness. The common types of hallucinogens are psychedelics, dissociatives and deliriants. Although hallucinations are a common symptom of amphetamine psychosis, amphetamines are not considered hallucinogens as they are not a primary effect of the drugs themselves. While hallucinations can occur when abusing stimulants, the nature of stimulant psychosis is not unlike delirium.

Nomenclature

A debate persists on criteria which would easily differentiate a substance which is 'psychedelic' from one 'hallucinogenic'.

A 'hallucinogen' and a 'psychedelic' may refer correctly to the same substance. Psychedelics are considered by many to be the 'traditional' or 'classical hallucinogens'. A 'hallucinogen' in this sense broadly refers to any substance which causes changes in perception or hallucinations, while psychedelics also carry a connotation of psychedelic culture.

Psychedelics (Classical Hallucinogens)

The word psychedelic was coined to express the idea of a drug that makes manifest a hidden but real aspect of the mind. It is commonly applied to any drug with perception-altering effects such as LSD and other ergotamine derivatives, DMT and other tryptamines including the alkaloids of *Psilocybe spp.* mescaline and other phenethylamines.

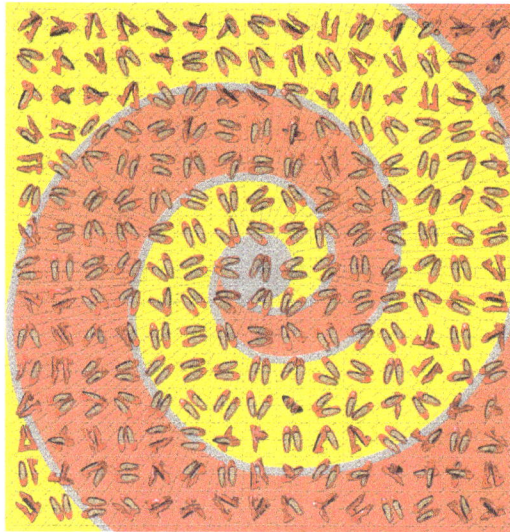

One "Blotter" sheet of 900 LSD doses.

The term psychedelic is applied somewhat interchangeably with psychotomimetic and hallucinogen, The classical hallucinogens are considered to be the representative psychedelics and LSD is generally considered the prototypical psychedelic. In order to refer to the LSD-like psychedelics, scientific authors have used the term "classical hallucinogen" in the sense defined by Glennon: "The classical hallucinogens are agents that meet Hollister's original definition, but are also agents that: (a) bind at 5-HT2 serotonin receptors, and (b) are recognized by animals trained to discriminate 1-(2,5-dimethoxy-4-methylphenyl)-2-aminopropane (DOM) from vehicle. Otherwise, when the term 'psychedelic' is used to refer only to the LSD-like psychedelics (a.k.a. the classical hallucinogens), authors explicitly point that they intend 'psychedelic' to be understood according to this more restrictive interpretation.

One explanatory model for the experiences provoked by psychedelics is the "reducing valve" concept. In this view, the drugs disable the brain's "filtering" ability to selectively prevent certain perceptions, emotions, memories and thoughts from ever reaching the conscious mind. This effect has been described as mind expanding, or consciousness expanding, for the drug "expands" the realm of experience available to conscious awareness.

While possessing a unique mechanism of action, cannabis or marijuana has historically been regarded alongside the classic psychedelics.

Research Chemicals and Designer Drugs

A designer drug is a structural or functional analog of a controlled substance that has been designed to mimic the pharmacological effects of the original drug while at the same time avoid being classified as illegal (by specification as a research chemical) and/or avoid detection in standard drug tests. Many designer drugs and research chemicals are hallucinogenic in nature, such as those in the 2C and 25-NB (NBOMe) families.

Dissociatives

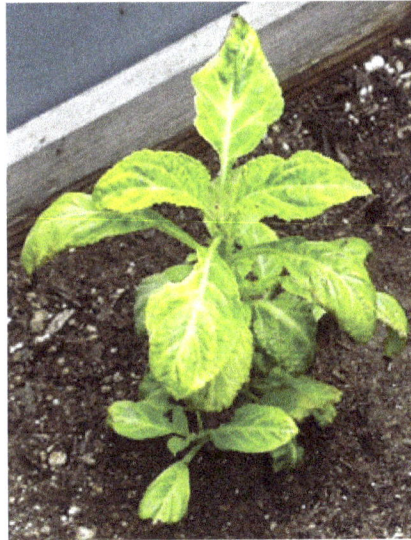

Salvia divinorum.

Dissociatives produce analgesia, amnesia and catalepsy at anesthetic doses. They also produce a sense of detachment from the surrounding environment, hence "the state has been designated as dissociative anesthesia since the patient truly seems disassociated from his environment." Dissociative symptoms include the disruption or compartmentalization of "the usually integrated functions of consciousness, memory, identity or perception." Dissociation of sensory input can cause derealization, the perception of the outside world as being dream-like or unreal. Other dissociative experiences include depersonalization, which includes feeling detached from one's body; feeling unreal; feeling able to observe one's actions but not actively take control;

being unable to recognize one's self in the mirror while maintaining rational awareness that the image in the mirror is the same person. Simeon offered "common descriptions of depersonalisation experiences: watching oneself from a distance (similar to watching a movie); candid out-of-body experiences; a sense of just going through the motions; one part of the self acting/participating while the other part is observing."

The classical dissociatives achieve their effect through blocking the signals received by the NMDA receptor set (NMDA receptor antagonism) and include ketamine, methoxetamine (MXE), phencyclidine (PCP), dextromethorphan (DXM), and nitrous oxide. However, dissociation is also remarkably administered by salvinorin A's (the active constituent in *Salvia divinorum* shown to the left) potent κ-opioid receptor agonism, though sometimes described as an atypical psychedelic.

Some dissociatives can have CNS depressant effects, thereby carrying similar risks as opioids, which can slow breathing or heart rate to levels resulting in death (when using very high doses). DXM in higher doses can increase heart rate and blood pressure and still depress respiration. Inversely, PCP can have more unpredictable effects and has often been classified as a stimulant and a depressant in some texts along with being as a dissociative. While many have reported that they "feel no pain" while under the effects of PCP, DXM and Ketamine, this does not fall under the usual classification of anesthetics in recreational doses (anesthetic doses of DXM may be dangerous). Rather, true to their name, they process pain as a kind of "far away" sensation; pain, although present, becomes a disembodied experience and there is much less emotion associated with it. As for probably the most common dissociative, nitrous oxide, the principal risk seems to be due to oxygen deprivation. Injury from falling is also a danger, as nitrous oxide may cause sudden loss of consciousness, an effect of oxygen deprivation. Because of the high level of physical activity and relative imperviousness to pain induced by PCP, some deaths have been reported due to the release of myoglobin from ruptured muscle cells. High amounts of myoglobin can induce renal shutdown.

Many users of dissociatives have been concerned about the possibility of NMDA antagonist neurotoxicity (NAN). This concern is partly due to William E. White, who claimed that dissociatives definitely cause brain damage. The argument was criticized on the basis of lack of evidence and White retracted his claim. White's claims and the ensuing criticism surrounded original research by John Olney.

In 1989, John Olney discovered that neuronal vacuolation and other cytotoxic changes ("lesions") occurred in brains of rats administered NMDA antagonists, including PCP and ketamine. Repeated doses of NMDA antagonists led to cellular tolerance and hence continuous exposure to NMDA antagonists did not lead to cumulative neurotoxic effects. Antihistamines such as diphenhydramine, barbiturates and even diazepam have been found to prevent NAN. LSD and DOB have also been found to prevent NAN.

Deliriants

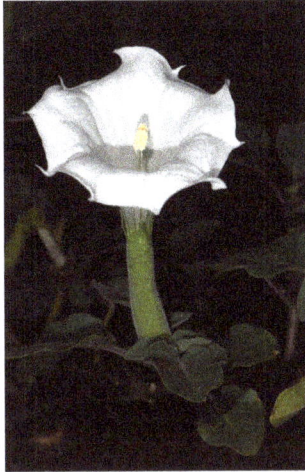

Datura

Deliriants, as their name implies, induce a state of delirium in the user, characterized by extreme confusion and an inability to control one's actions. They are called deliriants because their subjective effects are similar to the experiences of people with delirious fevers. The term was introduced by David F. Duncan and Robert S. Gold to distinguish these drugs from psychedelics and dissociatives, such as LSD and ketamine respectively, due to their primary effect of causing delirium, as opposed to the more lucid states produced by the other hallucinogens.

Despite the fully legal status of several common deliriant plants, deliriants are largely unpopular as recreational drugs due to the severe, generally unpleasant and often dangerous nature of the hallucinations produced.

Typical or classical deliriants are those which block the muscarinic acetylcholine receptors (antagonism). These are said to be anticholinergic. Many of these compounds are produced naturally in the nightshade plants, family Solanaceae. These tropane alkaloids are poisonous and can cause death due to tachycardia-induced heart failure and hyperthermia even in small doses. Additionally, over-the-counter antihistamines such as diphenhydramine (brand name Benadryl) and dimenhydrinate (brand name Dramamine) also have an anticholinergic effect. Uncured tobacco is also a deliriant due to its intoxicatingly high levels of nicotine.

The fly agaric mushroom, Amanita muscaria, is often informally lumped with the nightshade plants as a deliriant, though regarded as a dissociative with some regularity as well. This may be explained by the familiarity of both A. muscaria and Atropa belladonna to European culture, their formal statuses as deadly poisons, and their generally undesirable, unpleasant, and dangerous nature, with the potential for death from physical and behavioral toxicity a possibility even when dosages are carefully considered.

Nutmeg has deliriant and hallucinogenic effects as well due to some of its psychoactive chemicals, such as myristicin, which may be anticholinergic like the tropane alkaloids of the nightshade plants, or as suggested by Alexander Shulgin, partially metabolized into the empathogen-entactogen MMDA.

Psychedelics and Mental Illnesses in Long-term users

Most psychedelics are not known to have long-term physical toxicity. However, entactogens such as MDMA that release neurotransmitters may stimulate increased formation of free radicals possibly formed from neurotransmitters released from the synaptic vesicle. Free radicals are associated with cell damage in other contexts, and have been suggested to be involved in many types of mental conditions including Parkinson's disease, senility, schizophrenia, and Alzheimer's. Research on this question has not reached a firm conclusion. The same concerns do not apply to psychedelics that do not release neurotransmitters, such as LSD, nor to dissociatives or deliriants.

No clear connection has been made between psychedelic drugs and organic brain damage. However, hallucinogen persisting perception disorder (HPPD) is a diagnosed condition wherein certain visual effects of drugs persist for a long time, sometimes permanently, although science and medicine have yet to determine what causes the condition.

A large epidemiological study in the U.S. found that other than personality disorders and other substance use disorders, lifetime hallucinogen use was not associated with other mental disorders, and that risk of developing a hallucinogen use disorder was very low.

How Hallucinogens affect the Brain?

LSD, mescaline, psilocybin, and PCP are drugs that cause hallucinations, which can alter a person's perception of reality. LSD, mescaline, and psilocybin cause their effects by initially disrupting the interaction of nerve cells and the neurotransmitter serotonin. It is distributed throughout the brain and spinal cord, where the serotonin system is involved with controlling of the behavioral, perceptual, and regulatory systems. This also includes mood, hunger, body temperature, sexual behavior, muscle control, and sensory perception. Certain hallucinogens, such as PCP, act through a glutamate receptor in the brain which is important for perception of pain, responses to the environment, and learning and memory. Thus far, there have been no properly controlled research studies on the specific effects of these drugs on the human brain, but smaller studies have shown some of the documented effects associated with the use of hallucinogens.

Naming and Taxonomy

Psychedelic Nomenclature

Louis Lewin started out in 1928 by using the word phantastica as the title of his ground-breaking monograph about plants that, in his words, "bring about evident cerebral excitation in the form of hallucinations, illusions and visions followed by unconsciousness or other symptoms of altered cerebral functioning". But no sooner had the term been invented, or Lewin complained that the word "does not cover all that I should wish it to convey", and indeed with the proliferation of research following the discovery of LSD came numerous attempts to improve on it, such as hallucinogen, phanerothyme, psychedelic, psychotomimetic, psychogenic, schizophrenogenic, cataleptogenic, mysticomimetic, psychodysleptic, and entheogenic.

The word *psychotomimetic*, meaning "mimicking psychosis", reflects the hypothesis of early researchers that the effects of psychedelic drugs are similar to naturally occurring symptoms of schizophrenia, though it has since been discovered that some psychedelics resemble endogenous psychoses better than others. PCP and ketamine are known to better resemble endogenous psychoses because they reproduce both positive and negative symptoms of psychoses, while psilocybin and related hallucinogens typically produce effects resembling only the positive symptoms of schizophrenia. While the serotonergic psychedelics (LSD, psilocybin, mescaline, etc.) do produce subjective effects distinct from NMDA antagonist dissociatives (PCP, ketamine, dextrorphan), there is obvious overlap in the mental processes that these drugs affect and research has discovered that there is overlap in the mechanisms by which both types of psychedelics mimic psychotic symptoms. One double-blind study examining the differences between DMT and ketamine hypothesized that classically psychedelic drugs most resemble paranoid schizophrenia while dissociative drugs best mimicked catatonic subtypes or otherwise undifferentiated schizophrenia. The researchers expressed the view that "a heterogeneous disorder like schizophrenia is unlikely to be modeled accurately by a single pharmacological agent."

The word psychedelic was coined by Humphrey Osmond and has the rather mysterious but at least somewhat value-neutral meaning of "mind manifesting". The word entheogen, on the other hand, which is often used to describe the religious and ritual use of psychedelic drugs in anthropological studies, is associated with the idea that it could be relevant to religion. The words entactogen, empathogen, dissociative and deliriant, at last, have all been coined to refer to classes of drugs similar to the classical psychedelics that seemed deserving of a name of their own.

Many different names have been proposed over the years for this drug class. The famous German toxicologist Louis Lewin used the name phantastica earlier in this century, and as we shall see later, such a descriptor is not so farfetched. The most popular names—hallucinogen, psychotomimetic, and psychedelic ("mind manifesting")—have often been used interchangeably. Hallucinogen is now, however, the most common designation in the scientific literature, although it is an inaccurate descriptor of the actual effects of these drugs. In the lay press, the term psychedelic is still the most popular and has held sway for nearly four decades. Most recently, there has been a movement in nonscientific circles to recognize the ability of these substances to provoke mystical experiences and evoke feelings of spiritual significance. This term suggests that these substances reveal or allow a connection to the "divine within". Although it seems unlikely that this name will ever be accepted in formal scientific circles, its use has dramatically increased in the popular media and on internet sites. Indeed, in much of the counterculture that uses these substances, entheogen has replaced psychedelic as the name of choice and we may expect to see this trend continue.

Taxonomy

Hallucinogens can be classified by their subjective effects, mechanisms of action, and chemical structure. These classifications often correlate to some extent. In this topic, they are classified as psychedelics, dissociatives, and deliriants, preferably entirely to the exclusion of the inaccurate word hallucinogen, but the reader is well advised to consider that this particular classification is not universally accepted. The taxonomy used here attempts to blend these three approaches in order to provide as clear and accessible an overview as possible.

Almost all hallucinogens contain nitrogen and are therefore classified as alkaloids. THC and salvinorin A are exceptions. Many hallucinogens have chemical structures similar to those of human neurotransmitters, such as serotonin, and temporarily modify the action of neurotransmitters and/or receptor sites.

Leo Hollister's five criteria for establishing that a drug is hallucinogenic are as follows:

> "(1) In proportion to other effects, changes in thought, perception, and mood should predominate; (2) intellectual or memory impairment should be minimal; (3) stupor, narcosis, or excessive stimulation should not be an integral effect; (4) autonomic nervous system side effects should be minimal; and (5) addictive craving should be absent."

Lewin's Classes

A classical classification, mainly of historical interest, is that of Lewin:

> "*Class I Phantastica* roughly correspond to the psychedelics, which is a more modern term usually used as synonym to "hallucinogen" by people with positive attitudes towards them. Here the term is used a bit differently to discriminate one particular class of hallucinogens which it seems to describe best. They typically have no sedative effects (sometimes the opposite) and there is usually a clearcut memory to their effects. These drugs have also been referred to as the "classical" hallucinogens."

> "*Class II Phantastica* correspond to the other classes in our scheme. They tend to sedate in addition to their hallucinogenic properties and there often is an impaired memory trace after the effects wear off."

Pharmacological Classes of Hallucinogens

One possible way of classifying the hallucinogens is by their chemical structure and that of the receptors they act on. In this vein, the following categories are often used:

- Psychedelics:

    ◦ Serotonergics (5-HT_{2A} receptor agonists or classical psychedelics) such as mescaline from peyote (Lophophora williamsii):

        ▪ Indoles/Tryptamines such as psilocybin from "magic" mushrooms (Psilocybe).

        ▪ Ergolines such as lysergol from morning glory (Convolvulaceae).

        ▪ Lysergamides such as LSD ("acid"), derived from ergot (Claviceps purpurea).

        ▪ Beta-carbolines (monoamine oxidase inhibitors or MAOIs, specifically reversible inhibitors of monoamine oxidase A or RIMAs) such as harmala alkaloids such as norharman from ayahuasca (Banisteriopsis caapi).

        ▪ Complexly substituted tryptamines such as ibogaine from iboga (Tabernanthe iboga).

        ▪ Phenethylamines such as mescaline.

        ▪ Empathogen–entactogens such as MDA.

        ▪ Substituted methylenedioxyphenethylamines (serotonin releasing agents) such as MDMA ("ecstasy").

    ◦ Cannabinoidergics (CB-1 receptor agonists or atypical psychedelics) such as THC from cannabis (Cannabis).

- Dissociatives:

    ◦ Antiglutamatergics (NMDA receptor antagonists or classical dissociatives) such as "laughing gas" (nitrous oxide) and ketamine.

    ◦ Opioidergics (sometimes regarded as atypical psychedelics) (κ-Opioid receptor agonists or atypical dissociatives) such as salvinorin A from Salvia divinorum and pentazocine.

- Deliriants:

    ◦ Anticholinergics (muscarinic acetylcholine receptor antagonists or classical deliriants) such as tropane alkaloids such as atropine from deadly nightshade (*Atropa belladonna*) and diphenhydramine (Benadryl).

○   GABAergics (sometimes regarded as atypical dissociatives) ($GABA_A$ receptor agonists, and some positive allosteric modulators of the $GABA_A$ receptor, or atypical deliriants) such as muscimol from fly agaric (*Amanita muscaria*) and zolpidem (Ambien).

Problems with structure-based frameworks is that the same structural motif can include a wide variety of drugs which have substantially different effects. For example, both methamphetamine and MDMA are substituted amphetamines, but methamphetamine has a much stronger stimulant action than MDMA, with none of the latter's empathogenic effects. Also, drugs commonly act on more than one receptor; DXM, for instance, is primarily dissociative in high doses, but also acts as a serotonin reuptake inhibitor, similar to many phenethylamines.

Even so, in many cases structure-based frameworks are still very useful, and the identification of a biologically active pharmacophore and synthesis of analogues of known active substances remains an integral part of modern medicinal chemistry.

Recreational Drug Use

Recreational drug use is the use of a psychoactive drug to induce an altered state of consciousness for pleasure, by modifying the perceptions, feelings, and emotions of the user. When a psychoactive drug enters the user's body, it induces an intoxicating effect. Generally, recreational drugs are in three categories: depressants (drugs that induce a feeling of relaxation and calm); stimulants (drugs that induce a sense of energy and alertness); and hallucinogens (drugs that induce perceptual distortions such as hallucination). Many people also use prescribed and illegal opioids along with opiates and benzodiazepines. In popular practice, recreational drug use generally is a tolerated social behaviour, rather than perceived as the serious medical condition of self-medication. However, heavy use of some drugs is socially stigmatized.

Recreational drugs include alcohol (as found in beer, wine, and distilled spirits); cannabis (legal nationally in certain countries and state/province-wide or locally in others) and hashish; nicotine (tobacco); caffeine (coffee, tea, and soft drinks); prescription drugs; and the controlled substances listed as illegal drugs in the Single Convention on Narcotic Drugs and the Convention on Psychotropic Substances of the United Nations. What controlled substances are considered illegal drugs varies by country, but usually includes methamphetamine, heroin, cocaine, LSD, psilocybin mushrooms, MDMA and club drugs. In 2015, it was estimated that about 5% of people aged 15 to 65 had used illegal drugs at least once (158 million to 351 million).

Reasons for Use

Many researchers have explored the etiology of recreational drug use. Some of the most common theories are: genetics, personality type, psychological problems, self-medication, gender, age, instant gratification, basic human need, curiosity, rebelliousness, a sense of belonging to a group, family and attachment issues, history of trauma, failure at school or work, socioeconomic stressors, peer pressure, juvenile delinquency, availability, historical factors, or sociocultural influences. There has not been agreement around any one single cause. Instead, experts tend to apply the biopsychosocial model. Any number of these factors are likely to influence an individual's drug use as they are not mutually exclusive. Regardless of genetics, mental health or traumatic experiences, social factors play a large role in exposure to and availability of certain types of drugs and patterns of drug use.

According to addiction researcher Martin A. Plant, many people go through a period of self-redefinition before initiating recreational drug use. They tend to view using drugs as part of a general lifestyle that involves belonging to a subculture that they associate with heightened status and the challenging of social norms. Plant says, "From the user's point of view there are many positive reasons to become part of the milieu of drug taking. The reasons for drug use appear to have as much to do with needs for friendship, pleasure and status as they do with unhappiness or poverty. Becoming a drug taker, to many people, is a positive affirmation rather than a negative experience."

Evolution

Anthropological research has suggested that humans "may have evolved to counter-exploit plant neurotoxins". The ability to use botanical chemicals to serve the function of endogenous neurotransmitters may have improved survival rates, conferring an evolutionary advantage. A typically restrictive prehistoric diet may have emphasised the apparent benefit of consuming psychoactive drugs, which had themselves evolved to imitate neurotransmitters. Chemical–ecological adaptations, and the genetics of hepatic enzymes, particularly cytochrome P450, have led researchers to propose that "humans have shared a co-evolutionary relationship with psychotropic plant substances that is millions of years old."

Risks

Severity and type of risks that come with recreational drug use vary widely with the drug in question and the amount being used. There are many factors in the environment and within the user that interact with each drug differently. Overall, some studies suggest that alcohol is one of the most dangerous of all recreational drugs; only heroin, crack cocaine, and methamphetamines are judged to be more harmful. However, studies which focus on a moderate level of alcohol consumption have concluded that there can be substantial health benefits from its use, such as decreased risk of cardiac disease, stroke and cognitive decline. This claim has been disputed. Researcher David Nutt stated that these studies showing benefits for "moderate" alcohol consumption lacked control for the variable of what the subjects were drinking, beforehand. Experts in the UK have suggested that some drugs that may be causing less harm, to fewer users (although they are also used less frequently in the first place), include cannabis, psilocybin mushrooms, LSD, and ecstasy. These drugs are not without their own particular risks.

Responsible Use

The concept of "responsible drug use" is that a person can use drugs recreationally or otherwise with reduced or eliminated risk of negatively affecting other aspects of one's life or other people's lives. Advocates of this philosophy point to the many well-known artists and intellectuals who have used drugs, experimentally or otherwise, with few detrimental effects on their lives. Responsible drug use becomes problematic only when the use of the substance significantly interferes with the user's daily life.

Responsible drug use advocates that users should not take drugs at the same time as activities such as driving, swimming, operating machinery, or other activities that are unsafe without a sober state. Responsible drug use is emphasized as a primary prevention technique in harm-reduction drug policies. Harm-reduction policies were popularized in the late 1980s, although they began in the 1970s counter-culture, when cartoons explaining responsible drug use and the consequences of irresponsible drug use were distributed to users. Another issue is that the illegality of drugs in itself also causes social and economic consequences for those using them—the drugs may be "cut" with adulterants and the purity varies wildly, making overdoses more likely—and legalization of drug production and distribution would reduce these and other dangers of illegal drug use. Harm reduction seeks to minimize the harm that can occur through the use of various drugs, whether legal (e.g. alcohol and nicotine), or illegal (e.g. heroin and cocaine). For example, people who inject illicit drugs can minimize harm to both themselves and members of the community through proper injecting technique, using new needles and syringes each time, and proper disposal of all injecting equipment.

Prevention

In efforts to curtail recreational drug use, governments worldwide introduced several laws prohibiting the possession of almost all varieties of recreational drugs during the 20th century. The West's "War on Drugs" however, is now facing increasing criticism. Evidence is insufficient to tell if behavioral interventions help prevent recreational drug use in children.

One in four adolescents has used an illegal drug and one in ten of those adolescents who need addiction treatment get some type of care. School-based programs are the most commonly used method for drug use education despite the success rates of these intervention programs this success is highly dependent on the commitment of participants.

Demographics

Australia

Alcohol is the most widely used drug in Australia. 86.2% of Australians aged 12 years and over have consumed alcohol at least once in their lifetime, compared to 34.8% of Australians aged 12 years and over who have used cannabis at least once in their lifetime.

United States

In the 1960s, the number of Americans who had tried cannabis at least once increased over twentyfold. In 1969, the FBI reported that between the years 1966 and 1968, the number of arrests for marijuana possession, which had been outlawed throughout the United States under Marijuana Tax Act of 1937, had increased by 98%. Despite acknowledgement that drug use was greatly growing among America's youth during the late 1960s, surveys have suggested that only as much as 4% of the American population had ever smoked marijuana by 1969. By 1972, however, that number would increase to 12%. That number would then double by 1977.

The Controlled Substances Act of 1970 classified marijuana along with heroin and LSD as a Schedule I drug, i.e. having the relatively highest abuse potential and no accepted medical use. Most marijuana at that time came from Mexico, but in 1975 the Mexican government agreed to eradicate the crop by spraying it with the herbicide paraquat, raising fears of toxic side effects. Colombia then became the main supplier. The "zero tolerance" climate of the Reagan and Bush administrations resulted in passage of strict laws and mandatory sentences for possession of marijuana and in heightened vigilance against smuggling at the southern borders. The "war on drugs" thus brought with it a shift from reliance on imported supplies to domestic cultivation (particularly in Hawaii and California). Beginning in 1982, the Drug Enforcement Administration turned increased attention to marijuana farms in the United States, and there was a shift to the indoor growing of plants specially developed for small size and high yield. After over a decade of decreasing use, marijuana smoking began an upward trend once more in the early 1990s, especially among teenagers, but by the end of the decade this upswing had leveled off well below former peaks of use.

Society and Culture

Many movements and organizations are advocating for or against the liberalization of the use of recreational drugs, notably cannabis legalization. Subcultures have emerged among users of recreational drugs, as well as among those who abstain from them, such as teetotalism and "straight edge".

The prevalence of recreational drugs in human societies is widely reflected in fiction, entertainment, and the arts, subject to prevailing laws and social conventions. In video games, for example, enemies are often drug dealers, a narrative device that justifies the player killing them. Other games portray drugs as a kind of "power-up"; their effect is often unrealistically conveyed by making the screen wobble and blur.

Common Recreational Drugs

The following substances are used recreationally:

- Alcohol: Most drinking alcohol is ethanol, CH_3CH_2OH. Drinking alcohol creates intoxication, relaxation and lowered inhibitions. It is produced by the fermentation of sugars by yeasts to create wine, beer, and distilled liquor (e.g. vodka, rum, gin, etc.). In most areas of the world, it is legal for those over a certain age (18 in most countries). It is an IARC 'Group 1' carcinogen and a teratogen. Alcohol withdrawal can be life-threatening.

- Amphetamines: Used recreationally to provide alertness and a sense of energy. Prescribed for ADHD, narcolepsy, depression and weight loss. A potent central nervous system stimulant, in the 1940s and 50s methamphetamine was used by Axis and Allied troops in World War II, and, later on, other armies, and by Japanese factory workers. It increases muscle strength and fatigue resistance and improves reaction time. Methamphetamine use can be neurotoxic, which means it damages dopamine neurons. As a result of this brain damage, chronic use can lead to post acute withdrawal syndrome.

- Caffeine: Often found in coffee, black tea, energy drinks, some soft drinks (e.g. Coca-Cola, Pepsi and Mountain Dew, among others), and chocolate. It is the world's most widely consumed psychoactive drug, it has no dependence liability.

- Cannabis: Its common forms include marijuana and hashish, which are smoked or eaten. It contains at least 85 cannabinoids. The primary psychoactive component is THC, which mimics the neurotransmitter anandamide, named after the Hindu *ananda*, "joy, bliss, delight".

- Cocaine: It is available as a white powder, which is insufflated ("sniffed" into the nostrils) or converted into a solution with water and injected. A popular derivative, crack cocaine is typically smoked. When transformed into its freebase form, crack, the cocaine vapour may be inhaled directly. This is thought to increase bioavailability, but has also been found to be toxic, due to the production of methylecgonidine during pyrolysis.

- MDMA: Commonly known as ecstasy, it is a common club drug in the rave scene.

- Electronic cigarette: A large proportion of e-cigarette use is recreational. Most e-cigarette liquids contain nicotine, but the level of nicotine varies depending on user-preference and manufacturers. Nicotine is highly addictive, comparable to heroin or cocaine. E-cigarettes are being used to inhale MDMA, cocaine powder, crack cocaine, synthetic cathinones, mephedrone, α-PVP, synthetic cannabinoids, opioids, heroin, fentanyl, tryptamines, and ketamine.

- Ketamine: An anesthetic used legally by paramedics and doctors in emergency situations for its dissociative and analgesic qualities and illegally in the club drug scene.

- Lean: A liquid drug made when mixing cough syrup, sweets, soft drinks and codeine. It originated in the 1990s in Houston. Ever since then, this drug usage has grown and many people use this at parties becoming popular at the rave scene. Many people would get a drowsy feeling when consuming this drug.

- LSD: A popular ergoline derivative, that was first synthesized in 1938 by Hofmann. However, he failed to notice its psychedelic potential until 1943. In the 1950s, it was used in psychological therapy, and, covertly, by the CIA in Project MKULTRA, in which the drug was administered to unwitting US and Canadian citizens. It played a central role in 1960s 'counter-culture', and was banned in October 1968 by US President Lyndon B Johnson.

- Nitrous oxide: Legally used by dentists as an anxiolytic and anaesthetic, it is also used recreationally by users who obtain it from whipped cream canisters (whippets or whip-its), as it causes perceptual effects, a "high" and at higher doses, hallucinations.

- Opiates and opioids: Available by prescription for pain relief. Commonly abused opioids include oxycodone, hydrocodone, codeine, fentanyl, heroin, and morphine. Opioids have a high potential for addiction and have the ability to induce severe physical withdrawal symptoms upon cessation of frequent use. Heroin can be smoked, insufflated or turned into a solution with water and injected.

- Psilocybin mushrooms: This hallucinogenic drug was an important drug in the psychedelic scene. Until 1963, when it was chemically analysed by Albert Hofmann, it was completely unknown to modern science that *Psilocybe semilanceata* ("Liberty Cap", common throughout Europe) contains psilocybin, a hallucinogen previously identified only in species native to Mexico, Asia, and North America.

- Tobacco: *Nicotiana tabacum*. Nicotine is the key drug contained in tobacco leaves, which are either smoked, chewed or snuffed. It contains nicotine, which crosses the blood–brain barrier in 10–20 seconds. It mimics the action of the neurotransmitter acetylcholine at nicotinic acetylcholine receptors in the brain and the neuromuscular junction. The neuronal forms of the receptor are present both post-synaptically (involved in classical neurotransmission) and pre-synaptically, where they can influence the release of multiple neurotransmitters.

- Tranquilizers: Barbiturates, benzodiazepines (commonly prescribed for anxiety disorders; known to cause dementia and post acute withdrawal syndrome).

- "Bath salts": This is the street name for Mephedrone/Methylenedioxypyrovalerone (MDPV).

- DMT: Primary ingredient in ayahuasca, can also be smoked in a crack pipe; briefly (c. 30 minutes) causes a "total loss of connection to external reality".

- Peyote: This hallucinogen contains mescaline, native to southwestern Texas and Mexico.

- Salvia divinorum: This hallucinogenic Mexican herb in the mint family; not considered recreational, most likely due to the nature of the hallucinations (legal in some jurisdictions).

- Synthetic cannabis: Spice, K2, JWH-018, AM-2201.

- Research chemicals: 2C variants, etc.

Routes of Administration

Drugs often associated with a particular route of administration. Many drugs can be consumed in more than one way. For example, marijuana can be swallowed like food or smoked, and cocaine can be "sniffed" in the nostrils, injected, or, with various modifications, smoked.

- Inhalation: All intoxicative inhalants that are gases or solvent vapours that are inhaled through the trachea, as the name suggests.

- Insufflation: Also known as "sniffing", or "snorting", this method involves the user placing a powder in the nostrils and breathing in through the nose, so that the drug is absorbed by the mucous membranes. Drugs that are "sniffed", or "snorted", include powdered amphetamines, cocaine, heroin, ketamine and MDMA. Additionally, snuff tobacco.

- Intravenous Injection: The user injects a solution of water and the drug into a vein, or less commonly, into the tissue. Drugs that are injected include morphine and heroin, less commonly other opioids. Stimulants like cocaine or methamphetamine may also be injected. In rare cases, users inject other drugs.

- Oral Intake: Caffeine, ethanol, cannabis edibles, psilocybin mushrooms, coca tea, poppy tea, laudanum, GHB, ecstasy pills with MDMA or various other substances (mainly stimulants and psychedelics), prescription and over-the-counter drugs (ADHD and narcolepsy medications, benzodiazepines, anxiolytics, sedatives, cough suppressants, morphine, codeine, opioids and others).

- Sublingual: Substances diffuse into the blood through tissues under the tongue. Many psychoactive drugs can be or have been specifically designed for sublingual administration, including barbiturates, benzodiazepines, opioid analgesics with poor gastrointestinal bioavailability, LSD blotters, coca leaves, some hallucinogens. This route of administration is activated when chewing some forms of smokeless tobacco (e.g. dipping tobacco, snus).

- Intrarectal: Administering into the rectum, most water-soluble drugs can be used this way.

- Smoking: Tobacco, cannabis, opium, crystal meth, phencyclidine, crack cocaine and heroin (diamorphine as freebase) known as chasing the dragon.

- Transdermal patches with prescription drugs: e.g. methylphenidate (*Daytrana*) and fentanyl.

Many drugs are taken through various routes. Intravenous route is the most efficient, but also one of the most dangerous. Nasal, rectal, inhalation and smoking are safer. The oral route is one of the safest and most comfortable, but of little bioavailability.

Types

Depressants

Depressants are psychoactive drugs that temporarily diminish the function or activity of a specific part of the body or mind. Colloquially, depressants are known as "downers", and users generally take them to feel more relaxed and less tense. Examples of these kinds of effects may include anxiolysis, sedation, and hypotension. Depressants are widely used throughout the world as prescription medicines and as illicit substances. When these are used, effects may include anxiolysis (reduction of anxiety), analgesia (pain relief), sedation, somnolence, cognitive/memory impairment, dissociation, muscle relaxation, lowered blood pressure/heart rate, respiratory depression, anesthesia, and anticonvulsant effects. Depressants exert their effects through a number of different pharmacological mechanisms, the most prominent of which include facilitation of GABA or opioid activity, and inhibition of adrenergic, histamine or acetylcholine activity. Some are also capable of inducing feelings of euphoria (a happy sensation). The most widely used depressant by far is alcohol.

Stimulants or "uppers", such as amphetamines or cocaine, which increase mental or physical function, have an opposite effect to depressants.

Antihistamines

Antihistamines (or "histamine antagonists") inhibit the release or action of histamine. "Antihistamine" can be used to describe any histamine antagonist, but the term is usually reserved for the classical antihistamines that act upon the H_1 histamine receptor. Antihistamines are used as treatment for allergies. Allergies are caused by an excessive response of the body to allergens, such as the pollen released by grasses and trees. An allergic reaction causes release of histamine by the body. Other uses of antihistamines are to help with normal symptoms of insect stings even if there is no allergic reaction. Their recreational appeal exists mainly due to their anticholinergic properties, that induce anxiolysis and, in some cases such as diphenhydramine, chlorpheniramine, and orphenadrine, a characteristic euphoria at moderate doses. High dosages taken to induce recreational drug effects may lead to overdoses. Antihistamines are also consumed in combination with alcohol, particularly by youth who find it hard to obtain alcohol. The combination of the two drugs can cause intoxication with lower alcohol doses.

Hallucinations and possibly delirium resembling the effects of Datura stramonium can result if the drug is taken in much higher than therapeutical dosages. Antihistamines are widely available over the counter at drug stores (without a prescription), in the form of allergy medication and some cough medicines. They are sometimes used in combination with other substances such as alcohol. The most common unsupervised use of antihistamines in terms of volume and percentage of the total is perhaps in parallel to the medicinal use of some antihistamines to stretch out and intensify the effects of opioids and depressants. The most commonly used are hydroxyzine, mainly to stretch out a supply of other drugs, as in medical use, and the above-mentioned ethanolamine and alkylamine-class first-generation antihistamines, which are – once again as in the 1950s – the subject of medical research into their anti-depressant properties.

For all of the above reasons, the use of medicinal scopolamine for recreational uses is also seen.

Analgesics

Analgesics (also known as "painkillers") are used to relieve pain (achieve analgesia). Analgesic drugs act in various ways on the peripheral and central nervous systems; they include paracetamol (para-acetylaminophenol, also known in the US as acetaminophen), the nonsteroidal anti-inflammatory drugs (NSAIDs) such as the salicylates, and opioid drugs such as hydrocodone, codeine, heroin and oxycodone. Some further examples of the brand name prescription opiates and opioid analgesics that may be used recreationally include Vicodin, Lortab, Norco (hydrocodone), Avinza, Kapanol (morphine), Opana, Paramorphan (oxymorphone), Dilaudid, Palladone (hydromorphone), and OxyContin (oxycodone).

Tranquilizers

Tranquilizers (GABAergics):

- Barbiturates.

- Benzodiazepines.

- Ethanol (drinking alcohol; ethyl alcohol).

- Nonbenzodiazepines.

- Others:

  ◦ Carisoprodol (Soma).

  ◦ Chloral hydrate.

  ◦ Diethyl ether.

  ◦ Ethchlorvynol (Placidyl; "jelly-bellies").

- ○ Gamma-butyrolactone (GBL, a prodrug to GHB).

- ○ Gamma-hydroxybutyrate (GHB; G; Xyrem; "Liquid Ecstasy", "Fantasy").

- ○ Glutethimide (Doriden).

- ○ Kava (from *Piper methysticum*; contains kavalactones).

- ○ Ketamine.

- ○ Meprobamate (Miltown).

- ○ Methaqualone (Sopor, Mandrax; "Quaaludes").

- ○ Phenibut.

- ○ Propofol (Diprivan).

- ○ Theanine (found in *Camellia sinensis*, the tea plant).

- ○ Valerian (from *Valeriana officinalis*).

Stimulants

Stimulants, also known as "psychostimulants", induce euphoria with improvements in mental and physical function, such as enhanced alertness, wakefulness, and locomotion. Due to their effects typically having an "up" quality to them, stimulants are also occasionally referred to as "uppers". Depressants or "downers", which decrease mental or physical function, are in stark contrast to stimulants and are considered to be their functional opposites.

Stimulants enhance the activity of the central and peripheral nervous systems. Common effects may include increased alertness, awareness, wakefulness, endurance, productivity, and motivation, arousal, locomotion, heart rate, and blood pressure, and a diminished desire for food and sleep.

Use of stimulants may cause the body to significantly reduce its production of natural body chemicals that fulfill similar functions. Once the effect of the ingested stimulant has worn off the user may feel depressed, lethargic, confused, and miserable. This is referred to as a "crash", and may provoke reuse of the stimulant.

Examples include:

- Sympathomimetics (catecholaminergics)—e.g. amphetamine, methamphetamine, cocaine, methylphenidate, ephedrine, pseudoephedrine.

- Entactogens (serotonergics, primarily phenethylamines)—e.g. MDMA.

- Eugeroics, e.g. modafinil.

- Others:

  ◦ Arecoline (found in *Areca catechu*).

  ◦ Caffeine (found in *Coffea spp.*).

  ◦ Nicotine (found in *Nicotiana spp.*).

  ◦ Rauwolscine (found in *Rauvolfia serpentina*).

  ◦ Yohimbine (Procomil; a tryptamine alkaloid found in *Pausinystalia johimbe*).

Euphoriants

- Alcohol: Euphoria, the feeling of well-being, has been reported during the early (10–15 min) phase of alcohol consumption (e.g. beer, wine or spirits).

- Catnip: Catnip contains a sedative known as nepetalactone that activates opioid receptors. In cats it elicits sniffing, licking, chewing, head shaking, rolling, and rubbing which are indicators of pleasure. In humans, however, catnip does not act as a euphoriant.

- Cannabis: Tetrahydrocannabinol, the main psychoactive ingredient in this plant, can have sedative and euphoric properties.

- Stimulants: Psychomotor stimulants produce locomotor activity (the subject becomes hyperactive), euphoria, (often expressed by excessive talking and garrulous behaviour), and anorexia. The amphetamines are the best known drugs in this category.

- MDMA: The euphoriant drugs such as MDMA ('ecstasy') and MDEA ('eve') are popular among young adults. MDMA users experience short-term feelings of euphoria, rushes of energy and increased tactility.

- Opium: This drug derived from the unripe seed-pods of the opium poppy produces drowsiness and euphoria and reduces pain. Morphine and codeine are opium derivatives.

Hallucinogens

Hallucinogens can be divided into three broad categories: psychedelics, dissociatives, and deliriants. They can cause subjective changes in perception, thought, emotion and consciousness. Unlike other psychoactive drugs such as stimulants and opioids, hallucinogens do not merely amplify familiar states of mind but also induce experiences that differ from those of ordinary consciousness, often compared to non-ordinary forms of consciousness such as trance, meditation, conversion experiences, and dreams.

Psychedelics, dissociatives, and deliriants have a long worldwide history of use within medicinal and religious traditions. They are used in shamanic forms of ritual healing and divination, in initiation rites, and in the religious rituals of syncretistic movements such as União do Vegetal, Santo Daime, Temple of the True Inner Light, and the Native American Church. When used in religious practice, psychedelic drugs, as well as other substances like tobacco, are referred to as entheogens.

Starting in the mid-20th century, psychedelic drugs have been the object of extensive attention in the Western world. They have been and are being explored as potential therapeutic agents in treating depression, post-traumatic stress disorder, Obsessive-compulsive disorder, alcoholism, and opioid addiction. Yet the most popular, and at the same time most stigmatized, use of psychedelics in Western culture has been associated with the search for direct religious experience, enhanced creativity, personal development, and "mind expansion". The use of psychedelic drugs was a major element of the 1960s counterculture, where it became associated with various social movements and a general atmosphere of rebellion and strife between generations.

- Deliriants:
    - Atropine (alkaloid found in plants of the *Solanaceae* family, including datura, deadly nightshade, henbane and mandrake).
    - Dimenhydrinate (Dramamine, an antihistamine).
    - Diphenhydramine (Benadryl, Unisom, Nytol).
    - Hyoscyamine (alkaloid also found in the *Solanaceae*).
    - Hyoscine hydrobromide (another *Solanaceae* alkaloid).
    - Myristicin (found in *Myristica fragrans* ("Nutmeg")).
    - Ibotenic acid (found in *Amanita muscaria* ("Fly Agaric"); prodrug to muscimol).
    - Muscimol (also found in *Amanita muscaria*, a GABAergic).
- Dissociatives:
    - Dextromethorphan (DXM; Robitussin, Delsym, etc.; "Dex", "Robo", "Cough Syrup", "DXM").
    - Ketamine (K; Ketalar, Ketaset, Ketanest; "Ket", "Kit Kat", "Special-K", "Vitamin K", "Jet Fuel", "Horse Tranquilizer").
    - Methoxetamine (Mex, Mket, Mexi).
    - Phencyclidine (PCP; Sernyl; "Angel Dust", "Rocket Fuel", "Sherm", "Killer Weed", "Super Grass").

- ◦ Nitrous oxide (N_2O; "NOS", "Laughing Gas", "Whippets", "Balloons").

- • Psychedelics:

  - ◦ Phenethylamines.

    - ▪ 2C-B ("Nexus", "Venus", "Eros", "Bees").

    - ▪ 2C-E ("Eternity", "Hummingbird").

    - ▪ 2C-I ("Infinity").

    - ▪ 2C-T-2 ("Rosy").

    - ▪ 2C-T-7 ("Blue Mystic", "Lucky 7").

    - ▪ DOB.

    - ▪ DOC.

    - ▪ DOI.

    - ▪ DOM ("Serenity, Tranquility, and Peace" ("STP")).

    - ▪ MDMA ("Ecstasy", "E", "Molly", "Mandy", "MD", "Crystal Love").

    - ▪ Mescaline (found in peyote, Peruvian torch cactus and San Pedro cactus).

  - ◦ Tryptamines (including ergolines and lysergamides).

    - ▪ 5-MeO-DiPT ("Foxy", "Foxy Methoxy").

    - ▪ 5-MeO-DMT (found in various plants like chacruna, jurema, vilca, and yopo).

    - ▪ Alpha-methyltryptamine (αMT; Indopan; "Spirals").

    - ▪ Bufotenin (secreted by Bufo alvarius, also found in various Amanita mushrooms).

    - ▪ N,N-dimethyltryptamine (N,N-DMT; DMT; "Dimitri", "Disneyland", "Spice"; found in large amounts in Psychotria and in D. cabrerana).

    - ▪ Lysergic acid amide (LSA; ergine; found in morning glory and Hawaiian baby woodrose seeds).

    - ▪ Lysergic acid diethylamide (LSD; L; Delysid; "Acid", "Sid". "Cid", "Lucy", "Sidney", "Blotters", "Droppers", "Sugar Cubes").

    - ▪ Psilocin (found in psilocybin mushrooms).

- Psilocybin (also found in psilocybin mushrooms; prodrug to psilocin).

- Ibogaine (found in Tabernanthe iboga ("Iboga")).

- Atypicals:

  ◦ Salvinorin A (found in *Salvia divinorum*, a *trans*-neoclerodane diterpenoid ("Diviner's Sage", "Lady Salvia", "Salvinorin")).

Inhalants

Inhalants are gases, aerosols, or solvents that are breathed in and absorbed through the lungs. While some "inhalant" drugs are used for medical purposes, as in the case of nitrous oxide, a dental anesthetic, inhalants are used as recreational drugs for their intoxicating effect. Most inhalant drugs that are used non-medically are ingredients in household or industrial chemical products that are not intended to be concentrated and inhaled, including organic solvents (found in cleaning products, fast-drying glues, and nail polish removers), fuels (gasoline (petrol) and kerosene), and propellant gases such as Freon and compressed hydrofluorocarbons that are used in aerosol cans such as hairspray, whipped cream, and non-stick cooking spray. A small number of recreational inhalant drugs are pharmaceutical products that are used illicitly, such as anesthetics (ether and nitrous oxide) and volatile anti-angina drugs (alkyl nitrites).

The most serious inhalant abuse occurs among children and teens who "live on the streets completely without family ties". Inhalant users inhale vapor or aerosol propellant gases using plastic bags held over the mouth or by breathing from a solvent-soaked rag or an open container. The effects of inhalants range from an alcohol-like intoxication and intense euphoria to vivid hallucinations, depending on the substance and the dosage. Some inhalant users are injured due to the harmful effects of the solvents or gases, or due to other chemicals used in the products that they are inhaling. As with any recreational drug, users can be injured due to dangerous behavior while they are intoxicated, such as driving under the influence. Computer cleaning dusters are dangerous to inhale, because the gases expand and cool rapidly upon being sprayed. In some cases, users have died from hypoxia (lack of oxygen), pneumonia, cardiac failure or arrest, or aspiration of vomit.

Examples include:

- Chloroform,

- Ethyl chloride,

- Diethyl ether,

- Ethane and ethylene,

- Laughing gas (nitrous oxide),

- Poppers (alkyl nitrites),

- Solvents and propellants (including propane, butane, freon, gasoline, kerosene, toluene) and the fumes of glues containing them.

NEUROPSYCHOPHARMACOLOGY

Neuropsychopharmacology, an interdisciplinary science related to psychopharmacology (how drugs affect the mind) and fundamental neuroscience, is the study of the neural mechanisms that drugs act upon to influence behavior. It entails research of mechanisms of neuropathology, pharmacodynamics (drug action), psychiatric illness, and states of consciousness. These studies are instigated at the detailed level involving neurotransmission/receptor activity, bio-chemical processes, and neural circuitry. Neuropsychopharmacology supersedes psychopharmacology in the areas of "how" and "why", and additionally addresses other issues of brain function. Accordingly, the clinical aspect of the field includes psychiatric (psychoactive) as well as neurologic (non-psychoactive) pharmacology-based treatments. Developments in neuropsychopharmacology may directly impact the studies of anxiety disorders, affective disorders, psychotic disorders, degenerative disorders, eating behavior, and sleep behavior.

An implicit premise in neuropsychopharmacology with regard to the psychological aspects is that all states of mind, including both normal and drug-induced altered states, and diseases involving mental or cognitive dysfunction, have a neurochemical basis at the fundamental level, and certain circuit pathways in the central nervous system at a higher level. Thus the understanding of nerve cells or neurons in the brain is central to understanding the mind. It is reasoned that the mechanisms involved can be elucidated through modern clinical and research methods such as genetic manipulation in animal subjects, imaging techniques such as functional magnetic resonance imaging (fMRI), and in vitro studies using selective binding agents on live tissue cultures. These allow neural activity to be monitored and measured in response to a variety of test conditions. Other important observational tools include radiological imaging such as positron emission tomography (PET) and single-photon emission computed tomography (SPECT). These imaging techniques are extremely sensitive and can image tiny molecular concentrations on the order of 10^{-10} M such as found with extrastriatal D_1 receptor for dopamine.

One of the ultimate goals is to devise and develop prescriptions of treatment for a variety of neuropathological conditions and psychiatric disorders. More profoundly, though, the knowledge gained may provide insight into the very nature of human thought, mental abilities like learning and memory, and perhaps consciousness itself. A direct product of neuropsychopharmacological research is the knowledge base required to develop drugs which act on very specific receptors within a neurotransmitter system.

These "hyperselective-action" drugs would allow the direct targeting of specific sites of relevant neural activity, thereby maximizing the efficacy (or technically the *potency*) of the drug within the clinical target and minimizing adverse effects. However, there are some cases when some degree of pharmacological promiscuity is tolerable and even desirable, producing more desirable results than a more selective agent would. An example of this is Vortioxetine, a drug which is not particularly selective as a serotonin reuptake inhibitor, having a significant degree of serotonin modulatory activity, but which has demonstrated reduced discontinuation symptoms (and reduced likelihood of relapse) and greatly reduced incidence of sexual dysfunction, without loss in antidepressant efficacy.

The groundwork is currently being paved for the next generation of pharmacological treatments which will improve quality of life with increasing efficiency. For example, contrary to previous thought, it is now known that the adult brain does to some extent grow new neurons—the study of which, in addition to neurotrophic factors, may hold hope for neurodegenerative diseases like Alzheimer's, Parkinson's, ALS, and types of chorea. All of the proteins involved in neurotransmission are a small fraction of the more than 100,000 proteins in the brain. Thus there are many proteins which are not even in the direct path of signal transduction, any of which may still be a target for specific therapy. At present, novel pharmacological approaches to diseases or conditions are reported at a rate of almost one per week.

Neurotransmission

So far as we know, everything we perceive, feel, think, know, and do are a result of neurons firing and resetting. When a cell in the brain fires, small chemical and electrical swings called the action potential may affect the firing of as many as a thousand other neurons in a process called neurotransmission. In this way signals are generated and carried through networks of neurons, the bulk electrical effect of which can be measured directly on the scalp by an EEG device.

By the last decade of the 20th century, the essential knowledge of all the central features of neurotransmission had been gained. These features are:

- The synthesis and storage of neurotransmitter substances,

- The transport of synaptic vesicles and subsequent release into the synapse,

- Receptor activation and cascade function,

- Transport mechanisms (reuptake) and/or enzyme degradation.

The more recent advances involve understanding at the organic molecular level; biochemical action of the endogenous ligands, enzymes, receptor proteins, etc. The critical changes affecting cell firing occur when the signalling neurotransmitters from one neuron, acting as ligands, bind to receptors of another neuron. Many neurotransmitter systems and receptors are well known, and research continues toward the identification and characterization of a large number of very specific subtypes of receptors. For the six more important neurotransmitters Glu, GABA, Ach, NE, DA, and 5HT there are at least 29 major subtypes of receptor. Further "sub-subtypes" exist together with variants, totalling in the hundreds for just these 6 transmitters. It is often found that receptor subtypes have differentiated function, which in principle opens up the possibility of refined intentional control over brain function.

It has previously been known that ultimate control over the membrane voltage or potential of a nerve cell, and thus the firing of the cell, resides with the transmembrane ion channels which control the membrane currents via the ions K^+, Na^+, and Ca^{++}, and of lesser importance Mg^{++} and Cl^-. The concentration differences between the inside and outside of the cell determine the membrane voltage.

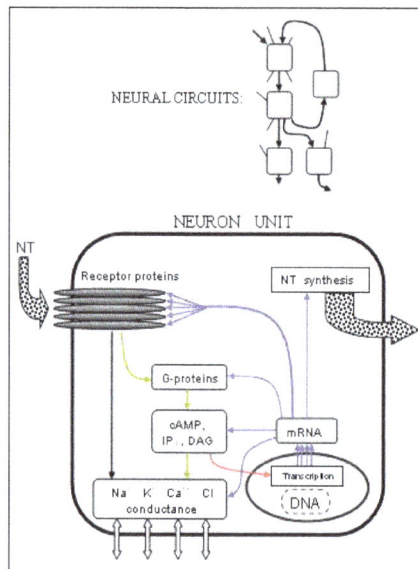

Abstract simplified diagram showing overlap between neurotransmission and metabolic activity. Neurotransmitters bind to receptors which cause changes to ion channels (black, yellow), metabotropic receptors also affect DNA transcription (red), transcription is responsible for all cell proteins including enzymes which manufacture neurotransmitters (blue).

Precisely how these currents are controlled has become much clearer with the advances in receptor structure and G-protein coupled processes. Many receptors are found to be pentameric clusters of five transmembrane proteins (not necessarily the same) or *receptor subunits*, each a chain of many amino acids. Transmitters typically bind at the junction between two of these proteins, on the parts that protrude from the cell membrane. If the receptor is of the ionotropic type, a central pore or channel in the middle of the proteins will be mechanically moved to allow certain ions to flow through, thus altering the ion concentration difference. If the receptor is of the metabotropic type, G-proteins will cause metabolism inside the cell that may eventually change other ion channels. Researchers are better understanding precisely how these changes occur based on the protein structure shapes and chemical properties.

The scope of this activity has been stretched even further to the very blueprint of life since the clarification of the mechanism underlying gene transcription. The synthesis of cellular proteins from nuclear DNA has the same fundamental machinery for all cells; the exploration of which now has a firm basis thanks to the Human Genome Project which has enumerated the entire human DNA sequence, although many of the estimated 35,000 genes remain to be identified. The complete neurotransmission process extends to the genetic level. Gene expression determines protein structures through type II RNA polymerase. So enzymes which synthesize or breakdown neurotransmitters, receptors, and ion channels are each made from mRNA via the DNA transcription of their respective gene or genes. But neurotransmission, in addition to controlling ion channels either directly or otherwise through metabotropic processes, also actually modulates gene expression. This is most prominently achieved through modification of the transcription initiation process by a variety of transcription factors produced from receptor activity.

Aside from the important pharmacological possibilities of gene expression pathways, the correspondence of a gene with its protein allows the important analytical tool of gene knockout. Living specimens can be created using homolog recombination in which a specific gene cannot be expressed. The organism will then be deficient in the associated protein which may be a specific receptor. This method avoids chemical blockade which can produce confusing or ambiguous secondary effects so that the effects of a lack of receptor can be studied in a purer sense.

Drugs

The inception of many classes of drugs is in principle straightforward: Any chemical that can enhance or diminish the action of a target protein could be investigated further for such use. The trick is to find such a chemical that is receptor-specific and safe to consume. The 2005 Physicians' Desk Reference lists twice the number of prescription drugs as the 1990 version. Many people by now are familiar with "selective serotonin reuptake inhibitors", or SSRIs which exemplify modern pharmaceuticals. These SSRI antidepressant drugs, such as Paxil and Prozac, selectively and therefore primarily inhibit the transport of serotonin which prolongs the activity in the synapse. There are numerous categories of selective drugs, and transport blockage is only one mode of action. The FDA has approved drugs which selectively act on each of the major neurotransmitters such as NE reuptake inhibitor antidepressants, DA blocker anti-psychotics, and GABA agonist tranquilizers (benzodiazepines).

New endogenous chemicals are continually identified. Specific receptors have been found for the drugs THC (cannabis) and GHB, with endogenous transmitters anandamide and GHB. Another recent major discovery occurred in 1999 when orexin, or hypocretin, was found to have a role in arousal, since the lack of orexin receptors mirrors the condition of narcolepsy. Orexin agonism may explain the antinarcoleptic action of the drug modafinil which was already being used only a year prior.

The next step, which major pharmaceutical companies are currently working hard to develop, are receptor subtype-specific drugs and other specific agents. An example is the push for better anti-anxiety agents (anxiolytics) based on $GABA_A(\alpha2)$ agonists, CRF_1 antagonists, and $5HT_{2c}$ antagonists. Another is the proposal of new routes of exploration for antipsychotics such as glycine reuptake inhibitors. Although the capabilities exist for receptor-specific drugs, a shortcoming of drug therapy is the lack of ability to provide anatomical specificity. By altering receptor function in one part of the brain, abnormal activity can be induced in other parts of the brain due to the same type of receptor changes. A common example is the effect of D_2 altering drugs (neuroleptics) which can help schizophrenia, but cause a variety of dyskinesias by their action on motor cortex.

Modern studies are revealing details of mechanisms of damage to the nervous system such as apoptosis (programmed cell death) and free-radical disruption. Phencyclidine has been found to cause cell death in striatopallidal cells and abnormal vacuolization in hippocampal and other neurons. The hallucinogen persisting perception disorder (HPPD), also known as post-psychedelic perception disorder, has been observed in patients as long as 26 years after LSD use. The plausible cause of HPPD is damage to the inhibitory GABA circuit in the visual pathway (GABA agonists such as midazolam can decrease some effects of LSD intoxication). The damage may be the result of an excitotoxic response of $5HT_2$ interneurons. Note that the vast majority of LSD users do not experience HPPD. Its manifestation may be equally dependent on individual brain chemistry as on the drug use itself. As for MDMA, aside from persistent losses of 5HT and SERT, long-lasting reduction of serotonergic axons and terminals is found from short-term use, and regrowth may be of compromised function.

Neural Circuits

It is a not-so-recent discovery that many functions of the brain are somewhat localized to associated areas like motor and speech ability. Functional associations of brain anatomy are now being complemented with clinical, behavioral, and genetic correlates of receptor action, completing the knowledge of neural signalling. The signal paths of neurons are hyperorganized beyond the cellular scale into often complex neural circuit pathways. Knowledge of these pathways is perhaps the easiest to interpret, being most recognizable from a systems analysis point of view, as may be seen in the following abstracts.

Almost all drugs with a known potential for abuse have been found to modulate activity (directly or indirectly) in the mesolimbic dopamine system, which includes and connects the ventral tegmental area in the midbrain to the hippocampus, medial prefrontal cortex, and amygdala in the forebrain; as well as the nucleus accumbens in the ventral striatum of the basal ganglia. In particular, the nucleus accumbens (NAc) plays an important role in integrating experiential memory from the hippocampus, emotion from the amygdala, and contextual information from the PFC to help associate particular stimuli or behaviors with feelings of pleasure and reward; continuous activation of this reward indicator system by an addictive drug can also cause previously neutral stimuli to be encoded as cues that the brain is about to receive a reward. This happens via the selective release of dopamine, a neurotransmitter responsible for feelings of euphoria and pleasure. The use of dopaminergic drugs alters the amount of dopamine released throughout the mesolimbic system, and regular or excessive use of the drug can result in a long-term downregulation of dopamine signaling, even after an individual stops ingesting the drug. This can lead the individual to engage in mild to extreme drug-seeking behaviors as the brain begins to regularly expect the increased presence of dopamine and the accompanying feelings of euphoria, but how problematic this is depends highly on the drug and the situation.

Significant progress has been made on central mechanisms of certain hallucinogenic drugs. It is at this point known with relative certainty that the primary shared effects of a broad pharmacological group of hallucinogens, sometimes called the "classical psychedelics", can be attributed largely to agonism of serotonin receptors. The $5HT_{2A}$ receptor, which seems to be the most critical receptor for psychedelic activity, and the $5HT_{2C}$ receptor, which is a significant target of most psychedelics but which has no clear role in hallucinogenesis, are involved by releasing glutamate in the frontal cortex, while simultaneously in the locus coeruleus sensory information is promoted and spontaneous activity decreases. $5HT_{2A}$ activity has a net pro-dopaminergic effect, whereas $5HT_{2C}$ receptor agonism has an inhibitory effect on dopaminergic activity, particularly in the prefrontal cortex. One hypothesis suggests that in the frontal cortex, $5HT_{2A}$ promotes late asynchronous excitatory postsynaptic potentials, a process antagonized by serotonin itself through $5HT_1$ receptors, which may explain why SSRIs and other serotonin-affecting drugs do not normally cause a patient to hallucinate. However, the fact that many classical psychedelics do in fact have significant affinity for $5HT_1$ receptors throws this claim into question. The head twitch response, a test used for assessing classical psychedelic activity in rodents, is produced by serotonin itself only in the presence of beta-Arrestins, but is triggered by classical psychedelics independent of beta-Arrestin recruitment. This may better explain the difference between the pharmacology of serotonergic neurotransmission (even if promoted by drugs such as SSRIs) and that of classical psychedelics. Newer findings, however, indicate that binding to the $5HT_{2A}$-mGlu2 heterodimer is also necessary for classical psychedelic activity. This, too, may be relevant to the pharmacological differences between the two. While early in the history of psychedelic drug research it was assumed that these hallucinations were comparable to those produced by psychosis and thus that classical psychedelics could serve as a model of psychosis, it is important to note that modern neuropsychopharmacological knowledge of psychosis has progressed significantly since then, and we now know that psychosis shows little similarity to the effects of classical psychedelics in mechanism, reported experience or most other respects aside from the surface similarity of "hallucination".

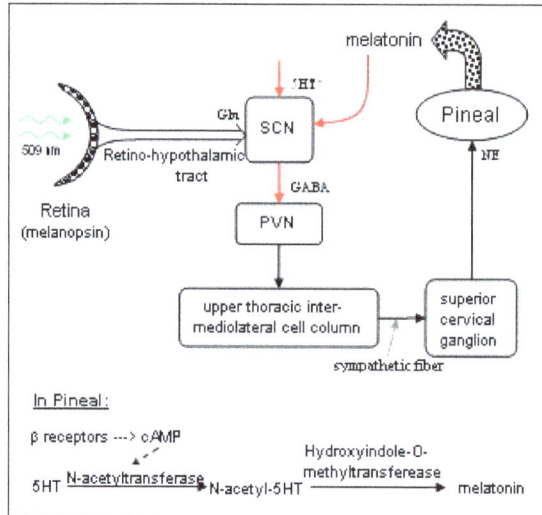

Diagram of neural circuit which regulates melatonin production via
actual circuit pathways. Green light in the eye inhibits pineal production of melatonin
(Inhibitory connections shown in red). Also shown: reaction sequence for melatonin synthesis.

Circadian rhythm, or sleep/wake cycling, is centered in the suprachiasmatic nucleus (SCN) within the hypothalamus, and is marked by melatonin levels 2000–4,000% higher during sleep than in the day. A circuit is known to start with melanopsin cells in the eye which stimulate the SCN through glutamate neurons of the hypothalamic tract. GABAergic neurons from the SCN inhibit the paraventricular nucleus, which signals the superior cervical ganglion (SCG) through sympathetic fibers. The output of the SCG, stimulates NE receptors (β) in the pineal gland which produces N-acetyltransferase, causing production of melatonin from serotonin. Inhibitory melatonin receptors in the SCN then provide a positive feedback pathway. Therefore, light inhibits the production of melatonin which "entrains" the 24-hour cycle of SCN activity. The SCN also receives signals from other parts of the brain, and its (approximately) 24-hour cycle does not only depend on light patterns. In fact, sectioned tissue from the SCN will exhibit daily cycle in vitro for many days. Additionally, the basal nucleus provides GABA-ergic inhibitory input to the pre-optic anterior hypothalamus (PAH). When adenosine builds up from the metabolism of ATP throughout the day, it binds to adenosine receptors, inhibiting the basal nucleus. The PAH is then activated, generating slow-wave sleep activity. Caffeine is known to block adenosine receptors, thereby inhibiting sleep among other things.

ROLE OF PSYCHOPHARMACOLOGY IN MENTAL HEALTH

Psychopharmacology has become a major approach to treatment in primary mental health disorders. However, combined psychiatric and medical illness can give rise to some challenging diagnostic problems. Furthermore, drug treatment of patients with such illnesses can involve important drug-disease interactions and drug-drug interactions. One should keep in mind the issues that arise when an emotionally troubled patient would benefit from a psychotropic drug but a concurrent medical illness complicates this treatment. An awareness of both the medical and psychiatric issues involved may make successful treatment possible. There is definitely a need for further research in the field, especially regarding major unresolved issues such as the proper selection of patients for whom antidepressants are indicated, clinical and biological predictors of treatment response, and the development of new treatments with superior efficacy and safety. Meanwhile, an empathic psychotherapeutic alliance coupled with careful clinical and pharmacological monitoring are the essential prerequisites for successful treatments.

IMPACT OF PSYCHOPHARMACOLOGY ON CONTEMPORARY PSYCHIATRY

Modern clinical psychopharmacology can be dated from the introduction of lithium carbonate to treat mania by John Cade in Australia in 1949 or from the introduction of chlorpromazine as the first synthetic drug found to be effective in both mania and psychotic disorders in Paris in the early 1950s. Soon thereafter, the mood-elevating effects of the monoamine oxidase inhibitor, iproniazid, and the antidepressant effects of imipramine were reported. By 1960, haloperidol, the first butyrophenone antipsychotic, the first so-called atypical antipsychotic, clozapine, and the benzodiazepines also were introduced. That is, at least one agent from each major class of currently employed psychotropic drugs was known by the end of the 1950s. These new treatments brought about fundamental changes in the treatment of many major psychiatric disorders of unknown cause—notably, mania, depression, acute and chronic psychotic disorders, including schizophrenia, as well as severe anxiety disorders. These changes can fairly be considered revolutionary. Moreover, their impact extended far beyond improvements in treatment, and included fundamental changes in the conceptualization of most psychiatric disorders, in their diagnosis and categorization, on models for research into the nature of psychiatric illnesses, on psychiatric education, on methods and standards for experimental therapeutics, and on the organization of modern psychiatry as a clinical and academic medical specialty.

In the first 2 decades of their introduction into psychiatric therapeutics, there was an intense struggle among the previous generation of psychiatrists who had been captivated by the psychodynamic and psychoanalytic tradition initiated by Sigmund Freud and his followers in the early 1900s. A common early assertion was that the new drugs might modify symptoms and limit pain and suffering, but left undone much of what was required to bring about major and sustained changes in behaviour and thinking. Nevertheless, a new generation of more medically or biologically oriented psychiatrists came to dominate psychiatry internationally, and to replace their more psychologically minded colleagues in positions of influence, including most university chairs of psychiatry.

Such sensitive questions arise as to whether the pharmacotherapeutic approach may have been overdone, with widespread degradation of standards for patient assessment and comprehensive care, as well as deeply affecting psychiatric education and the organization and functioning of psychiatric institutions and systems of care delivery. As noted by Dr David M Gardner and Dr Gustavo H Vázquez, there has appeared, in recent decades, a growing international inclination toward increasingly brief and routinized clinical encounters, with an emphasis on rapid but superficial diagnostic categorization and initiation of almost exclusively medicinal treatments. Even if such clinical practices were adequate, Dr Gardner emphasizes that they require extensive training, experience, knowledge, and judgment to be used effectively and safely. The argument can be made that heavy reliance on medicinal treatments with less emphasis on psychological approaches, and on symptom checklists rather than on thoughtful understanding of each patient has brought about fundamental changes in the theory and practice of modern psychiatry. These changes involve shifting the balance of tension between what has been labelled brainlessness versus mindlessness in psychiatry, in the biomedical direction. Such changes, in turn, are consistent with compelling efforts in recent decades to manage (limit) the costs of medical care of all types. Questions to be considered include whether this shift may be antithetical to comprehensive, thoughtful, and individualized care of people with psychiatric illness, and whether it provides an adequate model for psychiatric training.

Another profound effect of the introduction of effective and reasonably safe and tolerated medicinal treatments for psychiatric illnesses has been to reframe the tasks and possibilities for academic psychiatry and psychiatric research in a more biomedical perspective. This shift in interest was greatly stimulated by major technical and experimental advances that gave birth to the new field of neuroscience since the 1960s, culminating in recent explosive advances in structural and functional brain imaging, behavioural and neurogenetics, and molecular neuroscience. The changes in therapeutic practice as well as in research orientation marked a return to the 19th-century tradition of neuromedically oriented and descriptive psychiatry—a tradition that became neglected in the early-to-mid 20th century. A more biomedical approach is attractive, but may remain premature, and surely is an incomplete basis for understanding of most mental illnesses. As increasingly technically sophisticated and detailed information is developed in such fields as neuroimaging and neurogenetics, we are repeatedly reminded that almost all major mental disorders remain fundamentally idiopathic. Most lack not only known etiologies but also even a coherent pathophysiology. This fundamental truism limits efforts to develop a biomedically oriented psychiatry beyond the empirical application of psychotropics and detection of occasional coarse neurological disorders. Nevertheless, clinical and research efforts to develop a more biomedical psychiatry are appropriate and of great, but largely potential or even hypothetical, value. Indeed, the history of a series of movements in biology and medicine brought to address psychiatric disorders during the past 2 centuries is marked by time-limited enthusiasm, limited progress, and moving on to the next conceptual fashion. A point that is directly relevant to the present discussion of psychopharmacology is that the lack of a pathophysiology, let alone an etiology, for most psychiatric illnesses makes rational progress in therapeutics extremely difficult and highly risky from both a scientific and business perspective.

A fundamental aspect of the great leaps forward of psychopharmacology in the unprecedently innovative era of the 1950s is that nearly all of the discoveries of novel treatments and therapeutic theories rested not on rational prediction or laboratory experimentation arising from a secure pathological or pathophysiological basis, but largely on chance observations with immediate clinical implications—that is, the process of serendipity. Examples include the surprising clinical effects of lithium carbonate when used mainly for its putative anti-gout activity; observations, initially by surgeons and anesthesiologists, that chlorpromazine was not merely another sedative; unexpected mood changes in tuberculosis sanatoria on introduction of the N-isopropyl analog of isoniazid; surprising mood changes with imipramine, which looks chemically rather like another tricyclic antipsychotic; the counter-surprise that clozapine, though chemically rather imipraminelike, was not mood-elevating; and there are many others. A remarkable observation is that serendipity has not yet been replaced by modern neurobiology or advances in industrial or academic chemistry and neuropharmacology. Again, this conclusion follows from the lack of a tissue pathology or a plausible pathophysiology for most mental disorders.

A consequence of these circumstances is that there has been remarkably little fundamental innovation in psychopharmacologic therapeutics for psychiatry since the early 1960s. Most recently introduced psychotropics are modelled on chemical or pharmacodynamic similarities to earlier predecessors. This process has provided a viable business model and has led to patentable and often highly profitable new drug products, but very little that is fundamentally new or improved. In addition, psychotropic markets are saturating, patent protection is ending, and drug development pipelines are drying up. Indeed, there is a growing sense among pharmacological investigators and the pharmaceutical industry that we are stuck. In turn, a growing number of corporations are shifting investment and resources away from the central nervous system to apparently more tractable clinical problems that have indeed witnessed some striking and fundamental innovations in recent years. A consequence of the lack of innovation in psychotropic treatments, as emphasized by Dr Gardner, is that psychiatry is obliged to redouble efforts to make the best use of what we have while hoping for the next therapeutic breakthrough—whether guided by scientific theory or again through serendipity.

A further effect of the discovery of the several new classes of psychotropics in and following the 1950s is that a new kind of biological theorizing became dominant in academic psychiatry. The basic idea is that, as the science of drug action (pharmacodynamics) has made initial small advances, it has been irresistibly tempting to argue that the opposite of the drug action may be a clue to pathophysiology. Among other examples, this kind of thinking led to the dopamine-excess theory of psychotic disorders and mania based on the antidopaminergic actions of most antipsychoticantimanic drugs, to various monoamine deficiency hypotheses concerning depression and some anxiety disorders based on speculations about the norepinephrineor serotonin-potentiating actions of most antidepressants. Although such theorizing stimulated a generation of clever experimentation, findings of research aimed at testing them at the clinical level has remained inconsistent and unconvincing. This outcome should not be any more surprising than, for example, expecting to discover the pneumococcus from detailed knowledge of the molecular pharmacology of willow bark and its antipyretic salicylates. An extension of such speculations sometimes extends into clinical practice, as diagnoses or rationales for particular treatments are presented to patients couched in concepts arising from pharmacodynamics but representing little more than neuromythology. Again, the fundamental fact is that the disorders considered to lie within the province of psychiatry remain idiopathic.

The changes outlined above have had additional, fundamental effects on the theory and practice of psychiatry. One is that the shift away from 19th-century interests in a neurobiology of mental illness was also associated with a decline in interest in classic descriptive psychiatry and in psychopathology. This loss of interest largely continues, even in European centres where the tradition developed. It has also been accompanied by some peculiar developments in both psychiatric diagnosis and clinical practice. Regarding nosology, a former handful of credible psychiatric diagnoses has grown into a massive collection of hundreds of putative disorders to be found in standard international diagnostic manuals. Most of these are largely imperfectly defined and minimally investigated by traditional epidemiologic methods, continue to lack a coherent biology, and sometimes prove to be limited in clinical and research utility in the face of often complex or atypical clinical presentations. Examples include the highly unstable group of acute psychoses, most of which evolve into other disorders on follow-up, and the nearly incoherent group of major depressive disorders.

At the level of clinical practice, there is a strong temptation to simplify and generalize. To an antipsychotic, antidepressant, or mood-stabilizing hammer, many conditions look like nails. And yet, efforts to differentiate and optimize drug responses among clinical conditions or clinically defined types of patients remain primitive or ignored. Pressures to maintain broad, relatively nonspecific, markets for various types of psychotropics have been very high, as noted by Dr Vázquez. It has been tempting for both the pharmaceutical industry and psychiatric clinicians to ascribe great weight to findings of statistically significant improvements in randomized, placebo-controlled trials.

Indeed, the early years of modern psychopharmacology were at the forefront of development of current standard methods of design and analysis of controlled, clinical therapeutic trials. The problem is that most findings arise (quite appropriately) from trials designed to gain regulatory approval and to pursue the aims of a marketing plan, rather than to inform and refine rational clinical practice. Ironically, massive treasures of information about clinical subtypes of patients who did especially well or poorly with a given treatment, or tolerated it especially well or poorly, remain in computer banks held as proprietary information by pharmaceutical manufacturers, and left minimally evaluated by clinical investigators of all kinds. A far more sophisticated body of information is needed to inform and guide sound clinical practice. This information reasonably can include information on clinical subtypes and a more refined set of expectations of what a given treatment can reasonably be expected to do.

Dr Vázquez identifies additional factors that limit the ability of contemporary therapeutics research to contribute to a more sophisticated, specific, and predictable application of the available medicines that Dr Gardner challenges us to use more wisely. These include the tendency to generalize from averaged findings obtained with highly selected, often clinically unrepresentative, patient-subjects in therapeutic trials, and to make averages of averages in the currently enthusiastic application of data-pooling by the methods of meta-analysis. This kind of therapeutics research can usually identify useless or grossly intolerable compounds, but can hardly be expected to produce refined guidance for such basic clinical questions as which drug to start with and in what doses and for how long and for whom and then what? In addition to excessive generalization (for example, all forms of depression respond well and safely to antidepressants; antipsychotics are adequate treatment for all manifestations of schizophrenia), there is a tendency to overvalue or exaggerate the therapeutic efficacy of most psychotropics. In turn, such exaggerated expectations may arise from overvaluing probability values in comparisons of active drugs and placebos, rather than to attend to more relevant effect sizes (difference in drug, compared with placebo, response divided by variance of measurement).

Regarding such outcome measures, there is both good and bad news. Reassuring news includes findings of a recent, ambitious, and scholarly comparison of effect sizes of psychotropics to medicines employed in general medicine, which found relatively favourable results for many psychotropics. Not so good are clinically apparent tendencies to expect more of antipsychotics, antidepressants, mood stabilizers, or anxiolytics than they may deliver clinically with individual patients. Drug superiorities to placebo controls are typically in the range of 30% to 50%, often with impressive P values (which can be engineered to assure success of even a marginally effective treatment provided that the number of subjects is high). For example, antidepressants may average 30% to 40% higher rates of response than a randomly assigned placebo treatment, but such numbers can be misleading. Rarely do trial outcomes represent full clinical, symptomatic, or functional recovery. Instead, they typically involve changes in standardized rating scale scores (which may or may not be adequate surrogates for clinical assessment), usually aim for improvements as low as 50%, are carried out only for perhaps 6 or 8 weeks, and involve highly selected subjects who may not adequately represent clinically encountered patients with nominally similar diagnoses. Rather, similar averaged outcomes within any class of psychotropics are virtually inevitable as drugs would not be marketed if not superior to placebo in at least 2 (of sometimes numerous) trials. Indeed, it has proved difficult to demonstrate substantial, credible, and clinically meaningful differences between specific drugs within a given class in terms of efficacy and tolerability, whether they be antidepressants, anxiolytics, antipsychotics, or proposed mood stabilizers. Overall, despite their limitations, available averaged outcomes for most types of clinically employed psychotropics are generally favourable. Nevertheless, such evidence is far from being a sound basis on which to assume that the work of modern psychiatric therapeutics is simply to pick the right drug and an approximately appropriate dose for a given patient.

In addition, evidence for long-term effectiveness of most types of psychotropics in providing sustained benefits and protection from recurrences of psychiatric illnesses remains particularly limited and often based on ambiguous research methods. These include the potentially biasing selection of patients who respond, short term, to a given drug-product (whose manufacturer typically sponsors the trial) to continue (relatively briefly in comparison to the natural history of recurrence patterns) into aftercare that often involves randomized discontinuation to a placebo—that is, removing an apparently effective treatment, often with incomplete recovery from an acute illness. Such trial designs can add drug-discontinuation stress to factors associated with relapses or recurrences of illness, and so inflate apparent drug–placebo differences. Drug discontinuation can not only confound interpretation of long-term treatment trials but also sometimes have potentially dangerous, adverse effects on clinical treatment. Such risks are particularly evident in pregnancy, when many women and their physicians are more concerned with usually hypothetical or rare teratogenic effects than with common and major adverse effects on maternal health, and their unknown effects on the developing fetus.

A striking consequence arises from the evidently widely accepted belief that psychotropics routinely provide major clinical benefits and that a solution to most clinical problems can be found with the right drug or combination of drugs at the right doses. Such beliefs encourage what can be termed an allopathic compulsion to pursue pharmacological treatments relentlessly, uncritically, often rather thoughtlessly, and potentially dangerously. Moreover, given substantial risks of failure and high rates of partial or temporary symptomatic improvements with standard psychotropic treatments given in monotherapy, there is a growing temptation to try imaginative combinations or agents, higher than recommended doses, or to add unconventional treatments that lack regulatory approval for psychiatric applications. Most such practices appear to be responses to patient and clinician frustrations with lack of substantial clinical improvement. Even though some such efforts are often understandable, almost always, they lack specific scientific testing for added effectiveness with acceptable safety.

Given the appreciable limitations of modern psychotropic medicines to solve the complex human problems represented by most cases of psychiatric illness, it seems especially ironic that much of what psychiatry learned during the past 2 centuries—including efforts to develop descriptive nosologies, and psychopathological as well as psychodynamic understanding of people with psychiatric illness—appears to have become devalued in the competition with seemingly simple, effective, supposedly even sufficient, and certainly cost-effective, pharmacologically based treatments. This view of psychiatry is strongly encouraged by currently pervasive interest in savings of costs, time, and effort in this era of managed care. As has occurred with many previous movements in psychiatry (descriptive, psychopathological, neuromedical, psychodynamic, community psychiatry, and others), psychopharmacology is currently overvalued, and at long-term risk of being devalued or even abandoned, too. As noted by Dr Vázquez, an increasingly ominous trend in psychiatric clinical practice and in training programs, is the difficulty to engage in curiosity. The decline of curiosity has been encouraged by increasing pressures to produce more units of clinical product per hour, to save as much time and cost as possible, and to avoid asking questions that may seem to complicate understanding or care of a patient.

References

- Rose, Nikolas (2010). "Chapter 2 Historical changes in mental health practice". Historical changes in mental health practice. Oxford University Press. Doi:10.1093/med/9780199565498.003.0012. ISBN 9780199565498. Retrieved 24 April 2016

- What-is-Psychopharmacology, health: news-medical.net, Retrieved 28 June, 2019

- "FDA requires strong warnings for opioid analgesics, prescription opioid cough products, and benzodiazepine labeling related to serious risks and death from combined use". FDA. August 31, 2016. Retrieved 1 September 2016

- Role-of-psychopharmacology-in-mental-health, conferences-list: omicsonline.org, Retrieved 29 July, 2019

- Nelson, Max (2005). The Barbarian's Beverage: A History of Beer in Ancient Europe. Abingdon, Oxon: Routledge. P. 1. ISBN 0-415-31121-7. Retrieved 21 September 2010

- López-Muñoz, F.; Alamo, C. (2009). "Monoaminergic neurotransmission: the history of the discovery of antidepressants from 1950s until today". Current Pharmaceutical Design. 15 (14): 1563–1586. Doi:10.2174/138161209788168001. PMID 19442174

6

Diverse Fields in Pharmacology

There are various related fields of pharmacology. A few of them are pharmacoepidemiology, pharmacotoxicology, medicinal chemistry, pharmacogenomics and pharmacoinformatics. These diverse related fields of pharmacology have been thoroughly discussed in this chapter.

PHARMACOEPIDEMIOLOGY

Pharmacoepidemiology takes into consideration disciplines such as biostatistics, computer programming, epidemiology, administrative data, medicine, and pharmacology.

Organizations using Pharmacoepidemiology

Public health bodies, both national and global, are involved in pharmacoepidemiology. These health bodies include the World Health Organization (WHO), private sector organizations, and drug companies.

The Role of Pharmacovigilance

Pharmacovigilance, where the impact of a drug is monitored in populations using that particular product, is an integral aspect of pharmacoepidemiology. Organizations can track medicines for evidence of adverse events and safety issues as well as post-marketing activities. Similarly, having this long-term knowledge about a medicine and its impact can help scientists improve its use.

Pharmacoepidemiology came to the forefront in the 1960s when the use of antibiotics was being tracked in some European countries.

Also, pharmacoepidemiology was a useful tool when the thalidomide crisis occurred. Scientists noticed a rise in the percentage of abnormalities in infants born to women who were using thalidomide as a treatment for nausea. Pharmacoepidemiology was useful in this case for determining more information.

Pharmacoepidemiology Considerations

Pharmacoepidemiology uses clinical epidemiology to examine:

- Benefits and adverse effects.

- Drug-drug interactions for patients using more than one medicine.

- Medication non-adherence (when patients do not stick to the advised timings. and doses of medicines).

Researchers also need to be knowledgeable about the illness that the patients has to enable useful comparisons.

Another area that can be studied in depth is the profile of the doctors that are prescribing a type of medicine. Patterns in education, age, or gender may have an impact on how or what they prescribe.

Other aspects that may influence the use of specific medicines are the location of the doctor or whether the medic is more prone to being an early adopter for new medicines.

Reasons for Carrying out Pharmacoepidemiology

Post-marketing monitoring of a drug can help scientists discover the efficacy of the medicine as well as its toxicity. Cases of adverse events can be better tracked in the population through the use of pharmacoepidemiology.

Scientists can learn:

- The amount of cases of adverse events,

- How a medicine reacts with people who were not involved in previous studies,

- The impact of a medicine when combined with other drugs.

To generate an awareness of a drug's efficacy, heterogeneous groups of patients that share a similar age, gender, and comorbidities must be analyzed.

Researchers also have the opportunity to study the outcomes of a medicine in comparison to others on the market for the same disease. Examining a drug's use in the population can also reveal whether doctors are using the medicine for off-label treatments. With pharmacoepidemiology, scientists may also be able to deduce the impact of an overdose.

In addition to the health impact of a certain drug, economic details can be calculated for health bodies or governments. They can work out the cost per treatment day or the cost in relation to the patient's income.

PHARMACOTOXICOLOGY

Pharmacotoxicology entails the study of the consequences of toxic exposure to pharmaceutical drugs and agents in the health care field. The field of pharmacotoxicology also involves the treatment and prevention of pharmaceutically induced side effects. Pharmacotoxicology can be separated into two different categories: pharmacodynamics (the effects of a drug on an organism), and pharmacokinetics (the effects of the organism on the drug).

Mechanisms of Pharmaceutical Drug Toxicity

There are many mechanisms by which pharmaceutical drugs can have toxic implications. A very common mechanism is covalent binding of either the drug or its metabolites to specific enzymes or receptor in tissue-specific pathways that then will elicit toxic responses. Covalent binding can occur during both on-target and off-target situations and after biotransformation.

On-target Toxicity

On-target toxicity is also referred to as mechanism-based toxicity. This type of adverse effect that results from pharmaceutical drug exposure is commonly due to interactions of the drug with its intended target. In this case, both the therapeutic and toxic targets are the same. To avoid toxicity during treatment, many times the drug needs to be changed to target a different aspect of the illness or symptoms. Statins are an example of a drug class that can have toxic effects at the therapeutic target (HMG CoA reductase).

Immune Responses

Some pharmaceuticals can initiate allergic reactions, as in the case of penicillins. In some people, administration of penicillin can induce production of specific antibodies and initiate an immune response. Activation of this response when unwarranted can cause severe health concerns and prevent proper immune system functioning. Immune responses to pharmaceutical exposure can be very common in accidental contamination events. Tamoxifen, a selective estrogen receptor modulator, has been shown to alter the humoral adaptive immune response in gilthead seabream. In this case, pharmaceuticals can produce adverse effects not only in humans, but also in organisms that are unintentionally exposed.

Off-target Toxicity

Adverse effects at targets other than those desired for pharmaceutical treatments often occur with drugs that are nonspecific. If a drug can bind to unexpected proteins, receptors, or enzymes that can alter different pathways other than those desired for treatment, severe downstream effects can develop. An example of this is the drug eplerenone (aldosterone receptor antagonist), which should increase aldosterone levels, but has shown to produce atrophy of the prostate.

Bioactivation

Bioactivation is a crucial step in the activity of certain pharmaceuticals. Often times, the parent form of the drug is not the active form and it needs to be metabolized in order to produce its therapeutic effects. In other cases, bioactivation is not necessarily needed for drugs to be active and can instead produce reactive intermediates that initiate stronger adverse effects than the original form of the drug. Bioactivation can occur through the action Phase I metabolic enzymes, such as cytochrome P450 or peroxidases. Reactive intermediates can cause a loss of function in some enzymatic pathways or can promote the production of reactive oxygen species, both of which can increase stress levels and alter homeostasis.

Drug-drug Interactions

Drug-drug interactions can occur when certain drugs are administered at the same time. Effects of this can be additive (outcome is greater than those of one individual drug), less than additive (therapeutic effects are less than those of one individual drug), or functional alterations (one drug changes how another is absorbed, distributed, and metabolized). Drug-drug interactions can be of serious concern for patients who are undergoing multi-drug therapies. Coadministration of chloroquine, an anti-malaria drug, and statins for treatment of cardiovascular diseases has been shown to cause inhibition of organic anion-transporting polypeptides (OATPs) and lead to systemic statin exposure.

Pharmacotoxicity Examples

There are many different pharmaceutical drugs that can produce adverse effects after biotransformation, interaction with alternate targets, or through drug-drug interactions. All pharmaceuticals can be toxic, depending on the dose.

Acetaminophen

Acetaminophen (APAP) is a very common drug used to treat pain. High doses of acetaminophen has been shown to produce severe hepatotoxicity after being biotransformed to produce reactive intermediates. Acetaminophen is metabolized by CYP2E1 to produce NAPQI, which then causes significant oxidative stress due to increased reactive oxygen species (ROS). ROS can cause cellular damage in a multitude of ways, a few of which being DNA and mitochondrial damage and depletion of antioxidant enzymes such as glutathione. In terms of drug-drug interactions, acetaminophen activates CAR, a nuclear receptor involved in the production of metabolic enzymes, which increases the metabolism of other drugs. This could either cause reactive intermediates/drug activity to persist for longer than necessary, or the drug will be cleared quicker than normal and prevent any therapeutic actions from occurring. Ethanol induces CYP2E1 enzymes in the liver, which can lead to increased NAPQI formation in addition to that formed by acetaminophen.

Aspirin

Aspirin is an NSAID used to treat inflammation and pain. Overdoses or treatments in conjunction with other NSAIDs can produce additive effects, which can lead to increased oxidative stress and ROS activity. Chronic exposure to aspirin can lead to CNS toxicity and eventually affect respiratory function.

Anti-depressants

Anti-depressants have been prescribed since the 1950s, and their prevalence has significantly increased since then. There are many classes of anti-depressant pharmaceuticals, such as selective serotonin reuptake inhibitors (SSRIs), monoamine oxidase inhibitors (MAOIs), and tricyclic anti-depressants. Many of these drugs, especially the SSRIs, function by blocking the metabolism or reuptake of neurotransmitters to treat depression and anxiety. Chronic exposure or overdose of these pharmaceuticals can lead to seratonin and CNS hyperexcitation, weight changes, and, in severe cases, suicide.

Anti-cancer Drugs

Doxorubicin is a very effective anti-cancer drug that causes congestive heart failure while treating tumors. Doxorubicin is an uncoupling agent in that it inhibits proper functioning of complex I of the electron transport chain in mitochondria. It then leads to the production of ROS and the inhibition of ATP production. Doxorubicin has been shown to be selectively toxic to cardiac tissue, although some toxicity has been seen in other tissues as well. Other anti-cancer drugs, such as fluoropyrimidines and taxanes, are extremely effective at treating and reducing tumor proliferation, but have high incidences of cardiac arrhythmias and myocardial infarctions.

MEDICINAL CHEMISTRY

Medicinal chemistry and pharmaceutical chemistry are disciplines at the intersection of chemistry, especially synthetic organic chemistry, and pharmacology and various other biological specialties, where they are involved with design, chemical synthesis and development for market of pharmaceutical agents, or bio-active molecules (drugs).

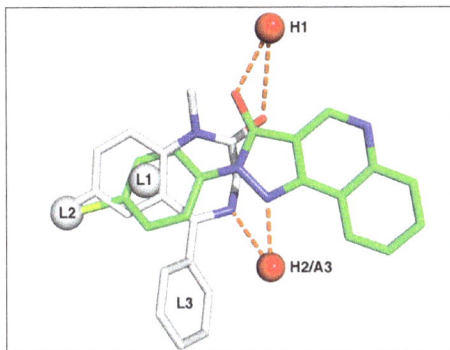

Medicinal chemistry seeks to develop therapeutic agents. Pharmacophore model of the benzodiazepine binding site on the GABAA receptor.

Compounds used as medicines are most often organic compounds, which are often divided into the broad classes of small organic molecules (e.g. atorvastatin, fluticasone, clopidogrel) and "biologics" (infliximab, erythropoietin, insulin glargine), the latter of which are most often medicinal preparations of proteins (natural and recombinant antibodies, hormones, etc.). Inorganic and organometallic compounds are also useful as drugs (e.g. lithium and platinum-based agents such as lithium carbonate and cisplatin as well as gallium).

In particular, medicinal chemistry in its most common practice—focusing on small organic molecules—encompasses synthetic organic chemistry and aspects of natural products and computational chemistry in close combination with chemical biology, enzymology and structural biology, together aiming at the discovery and development of new therapeutic agents. Practically speaking, it involves chemical aspects of identification, and then systematic, thorough synthetic alteration of new chemical entities to make them suitable for therapeutic use. It includes synthetic and computational aspects of the study of existing drugs and agents in development in relation to their bioactivities (biological activities and properties), i.e. understanding their structure-activity relationships (SAR). Pharmaceutical chemistry is focused on quality aspects of medicines and aims to assure fitness for purpose of medicinal products.

At the biological interface, medicinal chemistry combines to form a set of highly interdisciplinary sciences, setting its organic, physical, and computational emphases alongside biological areas such as biochemistry, molecular biology, pharmacognosy and pharmacology, toxicology and veterinary and human medicine; these, with project management, statistics, and pharmaceutical business practices, systematically oversee altering identified chemical agents such that after pharmaceutical formulation, they are safe and efficacious, and therefore suitable for use in treatment of disease.

In the Path of Drug Discovery

Discovery is the identification of novel active chemical compounds, often called "hits", which are typically found by assay of compounds for a desired biological activity. Initial hits can come from repurposing existing agents toward a new pathologic processes, and from observations of biologic effects of new or existing natural products from bacteria, fungi, plants, etc. In addition, hits also routinely originate from structural observations of small molecule "fragments" bound to therapeutic targets (enzymes, receptors, etc.), where the fragments serve as starting points to develop more chemically complex forms by synthesis. Finally, hits also regularly originate from *en-masse* testing of chemical compounds against biological targets, where the compounds may be from novel synthetic chemical libraries known to have particular properties (kinase inhibitory activity, diversity or drug-likeness, etc.), or from historic chemical compound collections or libraries created through combinatorial chemistry. While a number of approaches toward the identification and development of hits exist, the most successful techniques are based on chemical and biological intuition developed in team environments through years of rigorous practice aimed solely at discovering new therapeutic agents.

Hit to Lead and Lead Optimization

Further chemistry and analysis is necessary, first to identify the "triage" compounds that do not provide series displaying suitable SAR and chemical characteristics associated with long-term potential for development, then to improve remaining hit series with regard to the desired primary activity, as well as secondary activities and physiochemical properties such that the agent will be useful when administered in real patients. In this regard, chemical modifications can improve the recognition and binding geometries (pharmacophores) of the candidate compounds, and so their affinities for their targets, as well as improving the physicochemical properties of the molecule that underlie necessary pharmacokinetic/pharmacodynamic (PK/PD), and toxicologic profiles (stability toward metabolic degradation, lack of geno-, hepatic, and cardiac toxicities, etc.) such that the chemical compound or biologic is suitable for introduction into animal and human studies.

Process Chemistry and Development

The final synthetic chemistry stages involve the production of a lead compound in suitable quantity and quality to allow large scale animal testing, and then human clinical trials. This involves the optimization of the synthetic route for bulk industrial production, and discovery of the most suitable drug formulation. The former of these is still the bailiwick of medicinal chemistry, the latter brings in the specialization of formulation science (with its components of physical and polymer chemistry and materials science). The synthetic chemistry specialization in medicinal chemistry aimed at adaptation and optimization of the synthetic route for industrial scale syntheses of hundreds of kilograms or more is termed process synthesis, and involves thorough knowledge of acceptable synthetic practice in the context of large scale reactions (reaction thermodynamics, economics, safety, etc.). Critical at this stage is the transition to more stringent GMP requirements for material sourcing, handling, and chemistry.

Synthetic Analysis

The synthetic methodology employed in medicinal chemistry is subject to constraints that do not apply to traditional organic synthesis. Owing to the prospect of scaling the preparation, safety is of paramount importance. The potential toxicity of reagents affects methodology.

Structural Analysis

The structures of pharmaceuticals are assessed in many ways, in part as a means to predict efficacy, stability, and accessibility. Lipinski's rule of five focus on the number of hydrogen bond donors and acceptors, number of rotatable bonds, surface area, and lipophilicity. Other parameters by which medicinal chemists assess or classify their compounds are: synthetic complexity, chirality, flatness, and aromatic ring count.

PHARMACOGENOMICS

Pharmacogenomics is the study of the role of the genome in drug response. Its name (*pharmaco-* + *genomics*) reflects its combining of pharmacology and genomics. Pharmacogenomics analyzes how the genetic makeup of an individual affects his/her response to drugs. It deals with the influence of acquired and inherited genetic variation on drug response in patients by correlating gene expression or single-nucleotide polymorphisms with pharmacokinetics (drug absorption, distribution, metabolism, and elimination) and pharmacodynamics (effects mediated through a drug's biological targets). The term pharmacogenomics is often used interchangeably with pharmacogenetics. Although both terms relate to drug response based on genetic influences, pharmacogenetics focuses on single drug-gene interactions, while pharmacogenomics encompasses a more genome-wide association approach, incorporating genomics and epigenetics while dealing with the effects of multiple genes on drug response.

Pharmacogenomics aims to develop rational means to optimize drug therapy, with respect to the patients' genotype, to ensure maximum efficiency with minimal adverse effects. Through the utilization of pharmacogenomics, it is hoped that pharmaceutical drug treatments can deviate from what is dubbed as the "one-dose-fits-all" approach. Pharmacogenomics also attempts to eliminate the trial-and-error method of prescribing, allowing physicians to take into consideration their patient's genes, the functionality of these genes, and how this may affect the efficacy of the patient's current or future treatments (and where applicable, provide an explanation for the failure of past treatments). Such approaches promise the advent of precision medicine and even personalized medicine, in which drugs and drug combinations are optimized for narrow subsets of patients or even for each individual's unique genetic makeup. Whether used to explain a patient's response or lack thereof to a treatment, or act as a predictive tool, it hopes to achieve better treatment outcomes, greater efficacy, minimization of the occurrence of drug toxicities and adverse drug reactions (ADRs). For patients who have lack of therapeutic response to a treatment, alternative therapies can be prescribed that would best suit their requirements. In order to provide pharmacogenomic recommendations for a given drug, two possible types of input can be used: genotyping or exome or whole genome sequencing. Sequencing provides many more data points, including detection of mutations that prematurely terminate the synthesized protein (early stop codon).

Drug-Metabolizing Enzymes

There are several known genes which are largely responsible for variances in drug metabolism and response.

- Cytochrome P450s

- VKORC1

- TPMT

Cytochrome P450

The most prevalent drug-metabolizing enzymes (DME) are the Cytochrome P450 (CYP) enzymes. The term Cytochrome P450 was coined by Omura and Sato in 1962 to describe the membrane-bound, heme-containing protein characterized by 450 nm spectral peak when complexed with carbon monoxide. The human CYP family consists of 57 genes, with 18 families and 44 subfamilies. CYP proteins are conveniently arranged into these families and subfamilies on the basis of similarities identified between the amino acid sequences. Enzymes that share 35-40% identity are assigned to the same family by an Arabic numeral, and those that share 55-70% make up a particular subfamily with a designated letter. For example, CYP2D6 refers to family 2, subfamily D, and gene number 6.

From a clinical perspective, the most commonly tested CYPs include: CYP2D6, CYP2C19, CYP2C9, CYP3A4 and CYP3A5. These genes account for the metabolism of approximately 70-90% of currently available prescription drugs. The table below provides a summary for some of the medications that take these pathways.

Drug Metabolism of Major CYPs		
Enzyme	Fraction of drug metabolism (%)	Example Drugs
CYP2C9	10	Tolbutamide, ibuprofen, mefenamic acid, tetrahydrocannabinol, losartan, diclofenac.
CYP2C19	5	S-mephenytoin, amitriptyline, diazepam, omeprazole, proguanil, hexobarbital, propranolol, imipramine.

CYP2D6	20-30	Debrisoquine, metoprolol, sparteine, propranolol, encainide, codeine, dextromethorphan, clozapine, desipramine, haloperidol, amitriptyline, imipramine.
CYP3A4	40-45	Erythromycin, ethinylestradiol, nifedipine, triazolam, cyclosporine, amitriptyline, imipramine.
CYP3A5	<1	Erythromycin, ethinylestradiol, nifedipine, triazolam, cyclosporine, amitriptyline, aldosterone.

CYP2D6

Also known as debrisoquine hydroxylase (named after the drug that led to its discovery), CYP2D6 is the most well-known and extensively studied CYP gene. It is a gene of great interest also due to its highly polymorphic nature, and involvement in a high number of medication metabolisms (both as a major and minor pathway). More than 100 CYP2D6 genetic variants have been identified.

CYP2C19

Discovered in the early 1980s, CYP2C19 is the second most extensively studied and well understood gene in pharmacogenomics. Over 28 genetic variants have been identified for CYP2C19, of which affects the metabolism of several classes of drugs, such as antidepressants and proton pump inhibitors.

CYP2C9

CYP2C9 constitutes the majority of the CYP2C subfamily, representing approximately 20% of the liver content. It is involved in the metabolism of approximately 10% of all drugs, which include medications with narrow therapeutic windows such as warfarin and tolbutamide. There are approximately 57 genetic variants associated with CYP2C9.

CYP3A4 and CYP3A5

The CYP3A family is the most abundantly found in the liver, with CYP3A4 accounting for 29% of the liver content. These enzymes also cover between 40-50% of the current prescription drugs, with the CYP3A4 accounting for 40-45% of these medications. CYP3A5 has over 11 genetic variants identified at the time of this publication.

VKORC1

The vitamin K epoxide reductase complex subunit 1 (VKORC1) is responsible for the pharmacodynamics of warfarin. VKORC1 along with CYP2C9 are useful for identifying the risk of bleeding during warfarin administration. Warfarin works by inhibiting VKOR, which is encoded by the VKORC1 gene. Individuals with polymorphism in this have an affected response to warfarin treatment.

TPMT

Thiopurine methyltransferase (TPMT) catalyzes the S-methylation of thiopurines, thereby regulating the balance between cytotoxic thioguanine nucleotide and inactive metabolites in hematopoietic cells. TPMT is highly involved in 6-MP metabolism and TMPT activity and TPMT genotype is known to affect the risk of toxicity. Excessive levels of 6-MP can cause myelosuppression and myelotoxicity. Related patent litigation arose in Mayo Collaborative Services v. Prometheus Laboratories, Inc. in which the Supreme Court of the United States found that patent around measuring doses of the drug was patent-eligible.

Codeine, clopidogrel, tamoxifen, and warfarin a few examples of medications that follow the above metabolic pathways.

Predictive Prescribing

Patient genotypes are usually categorized into the following predicted phenotypes:

- Ultra-rapid metabolizer: Patients with substantially increased metabolic activity;

- Extensive metabolizer: Normal metabolic activity;

- Intermediate metabolizer: Patients with reduced metabolic activity;

- Poor metabolizer: Patients with little to no functional metabolic activity.

The two extremes of this spectrum are the poor metabolizers and ultra-rapid metabolizers. Efficacy of a medication is not only based on the above metabolic statuses, but also the type of drug consumed. Drugs can be classified into two main groups: active drugs and prodrugs. Active drugs refer to drugs that are inactivated during metabolism, and prodrugs are inactive until they are metabolized.

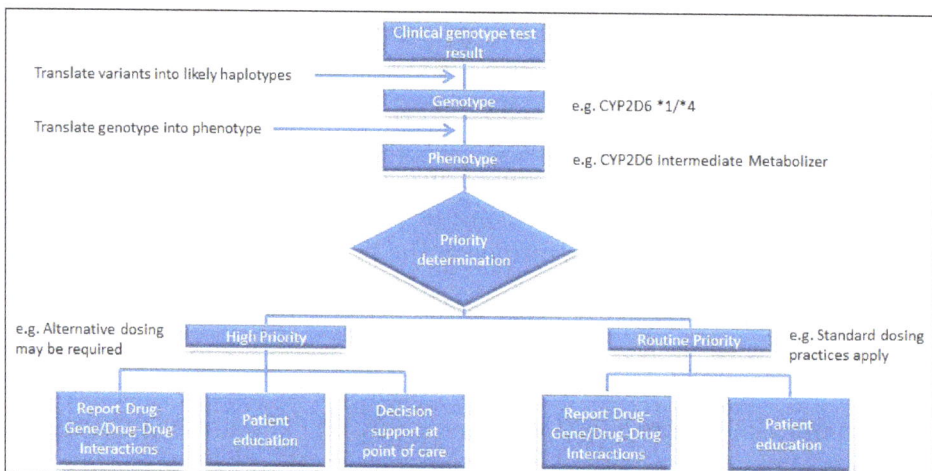

An overall process of how pharmacogenomics functions in a clinical practice. From the raw genotype results, this is then translated to the physical trait, the phenotype. Based on these observations, optimal dosing is evaluated.

For example, we have two patients who are taking codeine for pain relief. Codeine is a prodrug, so it requires conversion from its inactive form to its active form. The active form of codeine is morphine, which provides the therapeutic effect of pain relief. If person A receives one *1 allele each from mother and father to code for the CYP2D6 gene, then that person is considered to have an extensive metabolizer (EM) phenotype, as allele *1 is considered to have a normal-function (this would be represented as CYP2D6 *1/*1). If person B on the other hand had received one *1 allele from the mother and a *4 allele from the father, that individual would be an Intermediate Metabolizer (IM) (the genotype would be CYP2D6 *1/*4). Although both individuals are taking the same dose of codeine, person B could potentially lack the therapeutic benefits of codeine due to the decreased conversion rate of codeine to its active counterpart morphine.

Each phenotype is based upon the allelic variation within the individual genotype. However, several genetic events can influence a same phenotypic trait, and establishing genotype-to-phenotype relationships can thus be far from consensual with many enzymatic patterns. For instance, the influence of the CYP2D6*1/*4 allelic variant on the clinical outcome in patients treated with Tamoxifen remains debated today. In oncology, genes coding for DPD, UGT1A1, TPMT, CDA involved in the pharmacokinetics of 5-FU/capecitabine, irinotecan, 6-mercaptopurine and gemcitabine/cytarabine, respectively, have all been described as being highly polymorphic. A strong body of evidence suggests that patients affected by these genetic polymorphisms will experience severe/lethal toxicities upon drug intake, and that pre-therapeutic screening does help to reduce the risk of treatment-related toxicities through adaptive dosing strategies.

Applications

The list below provides a few more commonly known applications of pharmacogenomics:

- Improve drug safety, and reduce ADRs;

- Tailor treatments to meet patients' unique genetic pre-disposition, identifying optimal dosing;

- Improve drug discovery targeted to human disease;

- Improve proof of principle for efficacy trials.

Pharmacogenomics may be applied to several areas of medicine, including Pain Management, Cardiology, Oncology, and Psychiatry. A place may also exist in Forensic Pathology, in which pharmacogenomics can be used to determine the cause of death in drug-related deaths where no findings emerge using autopsy.

In cancer treatment, pharmacogenomics tests are used to identify which patients are most likely to respond to certain cancer drugs. In behavioral health, pharmacogenomic tests provide tools for physicians and care givers to better manage medication selection and side effect amelioration. Pharmacogenomics is also known as companion diagnostics, meaning tests being bundled with drugs. Examples include KRAS test with cetuximab and EGFR test with gefitinib. Beside efficacy, germline pharmacogenetics can help to identify patients likely to undergo severe toxicities when given cytotoxics showing impaired detoxification in relation with genetic polymorphism, such as canonical 5-FU. In particular, genetic deregulations affecting genes coding for DPD, UGT1A1, TPMT, CDA and CYP2D6 are now considered as critical issues for patients treated with 5-FU/ capecitabine, irinotecan, mercaptopurine/azathioprine, gemcitabine/capecitabine/ AraC and tamoxifen, respectively.

In cardiovascular disorders, the main concern is response to drugs including warfarin, clopidogrel, beta blockers, and statins. In patients with CYP2C19, who take clopidogrel, cardiovascular risk is elevated, leading to medication package insert updates by regulators. In patients with type 2 diabetes, haptoglobin (Hp) genotyping shows an effect on cardiovascular disease, with Hp2-2 at higher risk and supplemental vitamin E reducing risk by affecting HDL.

In psychiatry, as of 2010 research has focused particularly on 5-HTTLPR and DRD2.

Clinical Implementation

Initiatives to spur adoption by clinicians include the Ubiquitous Pharmacogenomics program in Europe and the Clinical Pharmacogenetics Implementation Consortium (CPIC) in the United States. In a 2017 survey of European clinicians, in the prior year two-thirds had not ordered a pharmacogenetic test.

In 2010, Valderbilt University Medical Center launched Pharmacogenomic Resource for Enhanced Decisions in Care and Treatment (PREDICT); in 2015 survey, two-thirds of the clinicians had ordered a pharmacogenetic test.

In the United States, the FDA has updated medication package inserts based on genomic evidence.

Case Studies

Case A – Antipsychotic adverse reaction.

Patient A suffers from schizophrenia. Their treatment included a combination of ziprasidone, olanzapine, trazodone and benzotropine. The patient experienced dizziness and sedation, so they were tapered off ziprasidone and olanzapine, and transition to quetiapine. Trazodone was discontinued. The patient then experienced excessive sweating, tachycardia and neck pain, gained considerable weight and had hallucinations. Five months later, quetiapine was tapered and discontinued, with ziprasidone re-introduction into their treatment due to the excessive weight gain. Although the patient lost the excessive weight they gained, they then developed muscle stiffness, cogwheeling, tremor and night sweats. When benztropine was added they experienced blurry vision. After an additional five months, the patient was switched from ziprasidone to aripiprazole. Over the course of 8 months, patient A gradually experienced more weight gain, sedation, developed difficulty with their gait, stiffness, cogwheel and dyskinetic ocular movements. A pharmacogenomics test later proved the patient had a CYP2D6 *1/*41, with has a predicted phenotype of IM and CYP2C19 *1/*2 with predicted phenotype of IM as well.

Case B – Pain Management.

Patient B is a woman who gave birth by caesarian section. Her physician prescribed codeine for post-caesarian pain. She took the standard prescribed dose, however experienced nausea and dizziness while she was taking codeine. She also noticed that her breastfed infant was lethargic and feeding poorly. When the patient mentioned these symptoms to her physician, they recommended that she discontinue codeine use. Within a few days, both the patient and her infant's symptoms were no longer present. It is assumed that if the patient underwent a pharmacogenomic test, it would have revealed she may have had a duplication of the gene CYP2D6 placing her in the Ultra-rapid metabolizer (UM) category, explaining her ADRs to codeine use.

Case C – FDA Warning on Codeine Overdose for Infants.

On February 20, 2013, the FDA released a statement addressing a serious concern regarding the connection between children who are known as CYP2D6 UM and fatal reactions to codeine following tonsillectomy and/or adenoidectomy (surgery to remove the tonsils and/or adenoids). They released their strongest Boxed Warning to elucidate the dangers of CYP2D6 UMs consuming codeine. Codeine is converted to morphine by CYP2D6, and those who have UM phenotypes are at danger of producing large amounts of morphine due to the increased function of the gene. The morphine can elevate to life-threatening or fatal amounts, as became evident with the death of three children in August 2012.

Polypharmacy

A potential role pharmacogenomics may play would be to reduce the occurrence of polypharmacy. It is theorized that with tailored drug treatments, patients will not have the need to take several medications that are intended to treat the same condition. In doing so, they could potentially minimize the occurrence of ADRs, have improved treatment outcomes, and can save costs by avoiding purchasing extraneous medications. An example of this can be found in psychiatry, where patients tend to be receiving more medications than even age-matched non-psychiatric patients. This has been associated with an increased risk of inappropriate prescribing.

The need for pharmacogenomics tailored drug therapies may be most evident in a survey conducted by the Slone Epidemiology Center at Boston University from February 1998 to April 2007. The study elucidated that an average of 82% of adults in the United States are taking at least one medication (prescription or nonprescription drug, vitamin/mineral, herbal/natural supplement), and 29% are taking five or more. The study suggested that those aged 65 years or older continue to be the biggest consumers of medications, with 17-19 % in this age group taking at least ten medications in a given week. Polypharmacy has also shown to have increased since 2000 from 23% to 29%.

Drug Labeling

The U.S. Food and Drug Administration (FDA) appears to be very invested in the science of pharmacogenomics as is demonstrated through the 120 and more FDA-approved drugs that include pharmacogenomic biomarkers in their labels. This number increased varies over the years. A study of the labels of FDA-approved drugs as of 20 June 2014 found that there were 140 different drugs with a pharmacogenomic biomarker in their label. Because a drug can have different biomarkers, this corresponded to 158 drug–biomarker pairs. Only 29% stated a requirement or recommendation for genetic biomarker testing but this was higher for oncology drugs (62%). Experts recognized the importance of the FDA's acknowledgement that pharmacogenomics experiments will not bring negative regulatory consequences.

Challenges

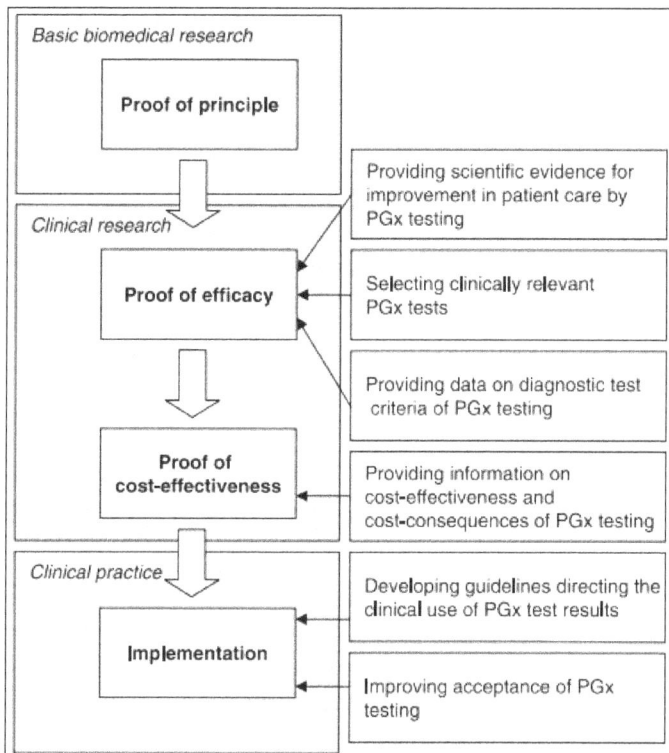

Consecutive phases and associated challenges in Pharmacogenomics.

Although there appears to be a general acceptance of the basic tenet of pharmacogenomics amongst physicians and healthcare professionals, several challenges exist that slow the uptake, implementation, and standardization of pharmacogenomics. Some of the concerns raised by physicians include:

- Limitation on how to apply the test into clinical practices and treatment;

- A general feeling of lack of availability of the test;

- The understanding and interpretation of evidence-based research; and

- Ethical, legal and social issues.

Issues surrounding the availability of the test include:

- The lack of availability of scientific data: Although there are considerable number of DME involved in the metabolic pathways of drugs, only a fraction have sufficient scientific data to validate their use within a clinical setting; and

- Demonstrating the cost-effectiveness of pharmacogenomics: Publications for the pharmacoeconomics of pharmacogenomics are scarce, therefore sufficient evidence does not at this time exist to validate the cost-effectiveness and cost-consequences of the test.

Although other factors contribute to the slow progression of pharmacogenomics (such as developing guidelines for clinical use), the above factors appear to be the most prevalent.

PHARMACOINFORMATICS

Pharmacoinformatics (or pharmacy informatics) is a sub-discipline of chemoinformatics involving the application of information technology in drug discovery and development. The field incorporates knowledge from numerous other disciplines, including bioinformatics, cancer informatics, immunoinformatics, neuroinformatics, and toxicoinformatics.

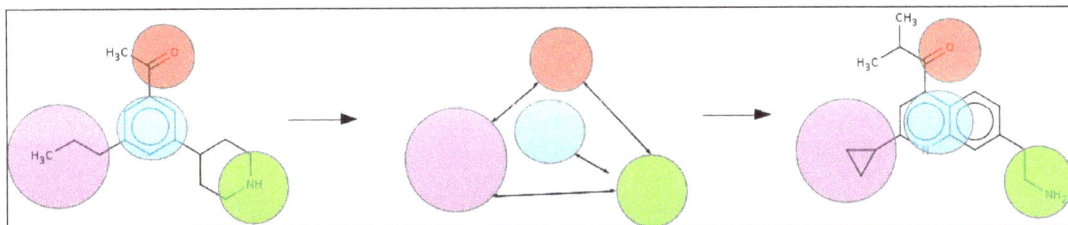

The creation of pharmacophores — models explaining how structurally diverse ligands can bind to a common receptor site — are used in virtual screening, which is vital to the field of pharmacoinformatics.

An alternate, more healthcare-related definition was suggested by the Healthcare Information and Management Systems Society (HIMSS) in 2007, describing pharmacoinformatics as "the scientific field that focuses on medication-related data and knowledge within the continuum of healthcare systems — including its acquisition, storage, analysis, use, and dissemination — in the delivery of optimal medication-related patient care and health outcomes."

Techniques and Tools

Virtual Screening

Virtual screening technology is vital to the field of pharmacoinformatics, with scientists heavily using it to computationally screen existing compound databases for hit/lead identifications rather than to conduct the actual molecular interaction and chemical research from scratch. In contrast to high-throughput screening, virtual screening involves computationally screening *in silico* libraries of compounds, by means of various methods such as docking, to identify members likely to possess desired properties such as biological activity against a given target. In some cases, combinatorial chemistry is used in the development of the library to increase the efficiency in mining the chemical space. More commonly, a diverse library of small molecules or natural products is screened. Such research often leads to positive results in the field of drug discovery; however, the process requires informatics tools to process data from virtual libraries, let alone store and organize them.

References

- Rodenas, M.C.; Cabas, I.; Abellán, E.; Meseguer, J.; Mulero, V.; García-Ayala, A. (December 2015). "Tamoxifen persistently disrupts the humoral adaptive immune response of gilthead seabream (Sparus aurata L.)". Developmental & Comparative Immunology. 53 (2): 283–292. Doi:10.1016/j.dci.2015.06.014

- What-is-Pharmacoepidemiology, health: news-medical.net, Retrieved 30 August, 2019

- U.S. Food and Drug Administration (FDA). "Table of Pharmacogenomic Biomarkers in Drug Labels". Retrieved 2014-09-03

- Pharmacoinformatics: limswiki.org, Retrieved 1 January, 2019

- Klaassen, Curtis D., ed. (2013). Casarett and Doull's toxicology : the basic science of poisons (8th ed.). New York: mcgraw-Hill Education. ISBN 978-0-07-176923-5

- Shin J, Kayser SR, Langaee TY (April 2009). "Pharmacogenetics: from discovery to patient care". Am J Health Syst Pharm. 66 (7): 625–37. Doi:10.2146/ajhp080170. PMID 19299369

Permissions

Index

www.ingramcontent.com/pod-product-compliance
Lightning Source LLC
Chambersburg PA
CBHW061953190326
41458CB00009B/2863